Multiple Choice Questions in

PHARMACOLOGY

Multiple Choice Questions in
PHARMACOLOGY

A. W. Bhagwat, MD., M.N.A.M.S., M.C.A.I.

Professor and Head, Department of Pharmacology
Medical College and Associated Hospital, Indore

New Central Book Agency (P) Ltd
8/1 Chintamoni Das Lane, Kolkata 700 009
India

Multiple Choice Questions in
PHARMACOLOGY

First Published : 2001
Reprinted : 2007

Publisher
New Central Book Agency (P) Ltd
8/1 Chintamoni Das Lane, Kolkata 700 009

Typesetter
Barun Sasmal
3 Garanhatta Street, Kolkata 700 006

Printer
New Central Book Agency (P) Ltd
Web-Offset Division, Dhulagarh, Sankrail, Howrah

Cover Designer
Ankit
6A Atalbehari Bose Lane, Kolkata 700 011

Technical Editor
Dr. Mita Sen, M.B.B.S.

Project Supervisor
Usha Ranjan Bhowmik

ISBN: 81-7381-396-5

Price : Rs. 135·00 [Rupees One Hundred and Thirty-five only]

Dedicated to

My wife Mrs. Asha,
Children Dr. (Mrs.) Anagha & Dr. Ashutosh
and
My Students

PREFACE

The material contained in these **Multiple Choice Questions** is not designed to provide the reader with an opportunity to escape from learning the basic information about the subject, which can only be obtained from a Standard Text Book of Pharmacology. The purpose of these MCQ's is to encourage the reader to detect areas of weakness in his understanding of the subject matter, so that he can return to his text for a more comprehensive study. While framing these questions it is presumed that the student has the basic knowledge about the subject and stress is given only on those aspects which the student is likely to miss or underestimate while going through the text, and which may form the basis for framing a question in an examination designed to eliminate students not suited for a given course of study e.g. Pre-P. G. and other competitive examinations. However, the questions will provide an interesting challange to the student and will give him an opportunity to improve his skills with multiple choice questions.

Author

CONTENTS

NOTE TO THE READERS

Reference 1 : BASIC AND CLINICAL PHARMACOLOGY [6th Ed., 1995]
B. G. Katzung

Reference 2 : THE PHARMACOLOGICAL BASIS OF THERAPEUTICS [9th Ed., 1996]
Goodman and Gillmans

Note

If in doubt the reader is advised to consult the page number(s) mentioned after each question of the Reference given at the beginning.

CHAPTER 1

AUTONOMIC NERVOUS SYSTEM

INSTRUCTIONS : FOR EACH OF THE FOLLOWING MULTIPLE CHOICE QUESTIONS SELECT THE BEST ANSWER

GENERAL

Reference 1

1. **Enteric nervous system is sometimes considered as :** 72
   a) A division of parasympathetic system
   b) A part of sympathetic system
   c) Third division of the Autonomic Nervous System
   d) Extension of somatic motor system

2. **The drug which blocks the transport of choline from extracellular fluid into the neuron, for the synthesis of Acetyl choline is :** 74
   a) Cocaine
   b) Hemicholinium
   c) Botulinum toxin
   d) Reserpine

3. **The transport of synthesised Acetyl choline from the cytoplasm into storage vesicle is blocked by :** 74
   a) Hemicholinium
   b) Reserpine
   c) Vesamicol
   d) Choline

4. **Botulinum toxin blocks :** 74
   a) Transport of acetyl choline into the storage vesicles
   b) Acetylation of choline
   c) Release of acetyl choline from vesicles by interacting with synaptobrevin
   d) Release of acetyl choline from vesicles by interacting with synaptotagmine

5. The rate limiting step in the synthesis of Noradrenaline is : 74

a) Transport of tyrosine into the neuron
b) Conversion of DOPA to dopamine
c) Conversion of tyrosine to DOPA
d) Conversion of DOPA to noradrenaline

6. The transport of dopamine into vesicles for conversion into noradrenaline is blocked by : 77

a) Cocaine
b) Guanethidine
c) Metyrosine
d) Reserpine

7. The release of noradrenaline from nerve terminal is blocked by : 77

a) Bretyllium
b) Reserpine
c) Verapamil
d) Cocaine

8. The transport of released noradrenaline back into cytoplasm (Uptake I) is blocked by : 77

a) Cocaine
b) Reserpine
c) Bretylium
d) Tricyclic antidepressants
e) By drugs a and c
f) By drugs a and d

9. The enzyme tyrosine hydroxylase which converts tyrosin into DOPA is inhibited by : 74

a) Physostigmine
b) Pyragalol
c) Metyrosin
d) Tranylcypromine

10. Following adrenergic nerve stimulation, the release of noradrenaline is accompanied by the release of : 74

a) Acetyl choline, ATP and peptide cotransmitters
b) ATP, dopamine-beta-hydroxylase and peptide cotransmitters
c) Tyrosine hydroxylase, ATP and calcium
d) ATP, dopamine, tyrosine and dopamine-beta-hydroxylase

11. Neurotransmitters identified in the nonadrenergic, noncholinergic neurons present in the autonomic effector tissues include all of the following EXCEPT : 76

a) ATP
b) Neuropeptide Y
c) Cholecystokinin
d) Serotonin
e) Histamine

12. **The Drug which can cause release of transmitter from nonadrenergic, noncholinergic neurons is :** 79

a) Calcium
b) Capsaicin
c) ADP
d) Neostigmine

13. **Explosive release of transmitter from adrenergic and cholinergic vesicles is caused by :** 84

a) Tyramine
b) Conotoxin
c) Latrotoxin
d) Nicotine
e) Botulinum toxin

14. **Presynaptic receptors which respond to the transmitter released from the nerve endings have been called as :** 83

a) Heteroreceptors
b) Homoreceptors
c) Autoreceptors
d) Baroreceptors

15. **Adrenergic nerve terminals are destroyed by which of the following drug :** 84

a) Reserpine
b) Tyramine
c) Tetrodoxin
d) 6-Hydroxydopamine
e) Metyrosine

Reference 2

16. **Which of the following drug blocks axonal conduction by blocking the voltage sensitive Sodium channel :** 112

a) Hemicholinium
b) Vesamicol
c) Tetrodotoxin
d) Bugarotoxin

17. **The drug which blocks axonal conduction by causing persistent depolarisation is :** 112

a) Saxitoxin
b) Botulinum toxin
c) Syntaxin
d) Batrachotoxin
e) Amotoxin

18. **Which of the following drug inhibits release of norepinephrine by interaction with specific presynaptic receptors :** 114

a) Clonidine

b) Adenosine
c) Acetylcholine
d) Dopamine
e) Prostaglandins
f) All of the above

19. **The most important mechanism involved in terminating the action of norepinephrine is :** 114
a) Destruction by MAO
b) Destruction by COMT
c) Diffusion across the synaptic cleft and reuptake by adrenergic neurons
d) All of the above

20. **The rate limiting step in the synthesis of acetyl choline is :** 115
a) Acetylation of choline
b) Uptake of choline by neurons
c) Formation of Acetyl coenzyme A
d) Formation of Acetyl AMP

ANSWERS

1.c 2.b 3.c 4.c 5.c 6.d 7.a 8.f 9.c 10.b 11.e 12.b 13.c 14.c 15.d 16.c 17.d 18.f 19.c 20.b

CHOLINOMIMETIC DRUGS

Reference 1

21. **Activation of muscarinic receptors results in all of the following EXCEPT :** 89
a) Activation of IP3,DAG cascade
b) Inhibition of adenyl cyclase activity
c) Increased cellular concentration of cyclic GMP
d) Increased cellular concentration of cyclic AMP
e) Opening of potassium channels

22. **Activation of Nicotinic receptors results in :** 88
a) Stimulation of adenyl cyclase activity
b) Opening of cation selective ion channels
c) Increased concentration of diacylglycerol
d) Increased concentration of cyclic AMP and GMP

23. **Musacrinic receptors present in the heart are labelled as :** 89
a) M-1 receptors
b) M-3 receptors
c) M-2 receptors
d) None of these

24. **Choline ester which possesses only muscarinic action and is resistant to destruction by cholinesterase is :** 91
a) Neostigmine

b) Physostigmine
c) Carbachol
d) Bethanicol
e) Mecholyl

25. **The most potent muscarinic agonist is :** 90
a) Carbachol
b) Methacholine
c) Neostigmine
d) Muscarine
e) Oxotremorine

26. **Dimethylphenylpiperazinium is a drug which is used as a research tool for selective stimulation of :** 90
a) Muscarinic receptors
b) Adenosine receptors
c) Serotonin receptors
d) Ganglionic Nicotinic receptors
e) Neuromuscular Nicotinic receptors

27. **The drug used as a marker for Nicotinic receptors is :** 92
a) Latrotoxin
b) Alpha-Bugarotoxin
c) Conotoxin
d) Capsaicin

28. **The distribution of Cholinoceptors in the CNS is as :** 93
a) Brain is richer in muscarinic sites and spinal cord in nicotinic sites
b) Brain is richer in nicotinic sites and spinal cord in muscarinic sites
c) Brain and spinal cord have equal number of muscarinic and nicotinic sites
d) There are no muscarinic receptors in either brain or spinal cord

29. **Echothiophate is the preferred irreversible cholinesterase inhibitor for clinical use because :** 94
a) It acts very rapidly
b) It has long duration of action and is stable in aqueous solution
c) It is the least toxic of all the organophosphates
d) It is highly lipid-soluble and hence penetrates tissues better

30. **The thiophosphate which is inactive as such and is converted into active phosphate insecticide derivative in animals and plants is :** 94
a) DFP
b) TEPP
c) OMPA
d) Malathion

31. **The shortest acting anticholinesterase drug is :** 96
a) Neostigmine
b) Physostigmine
c) Pyridostigmine

d) Ambenonium
e) Endrophonium

32. **Cardiovascular effects of cholinesterase inhibitors include all of the following EXCEPT :** 97
a) Decreased heart rate
b) Dilatation of blood vessels
c) Blockade of conduction through A-V junction
d) Diminished atrial contractility

33. **Therapeutic indications of the cholinomimetic drugs include all of the following EXCEPT :** 99
a) Glaucoma
b) GIT atony
c) Myasthenia gravis
d) Supraventricular tachycardia
e) Urinary retention

34. **Cholinomimetic drug preferred for the treatment of Alzheimer's disease is :** 97
a) Tacrine
b) Physostigmine
c) Pyridostigmine
d) Demecarinium

35. **Cholinesterase inhibitors reduce intraocular pressure in glaucoma by :** 98
a) Decreasing the formation of aqueous humor
b) Facilitating the outflow of aqueous humor
c) Drawing fluid from the eye by an osmotic effect
d) Facilitating outflow of aqueous humor and also diminishing its rate of secretion.

36. **The drug used to differentiate between myasthenic crisis and cholinergic crisis is :** 99
a) Neostigmine
b) Pyridostigmine
c) Acetyl choline
d) Endrophonium

37. **Longer acting cholinesterase inhibitors are not used for the long term treatment of Myasthenia gravis because :** 99
a) They are difficult to administer and self-medication is not possible
b) Dose requirement in this disease changes too rapidly to permit smooth control
c) They are too toxic for prolonged use
d) Their effect on the neuromuscular junction is variable

38. **The drug of choice for the treatment of supraventricular tachycardia is :** 99
a) Mecholyl
b) Carbachol
c) Adenosin
d) Endrophonium
e) Neostigmine

ANSWERS

21.d 22.b 23.c 24.d 25.e 26.d 27.b 28.a 29.b 30.d 31.e 32.b 33.d 34.a 35.d 36.d 37.b 38.c

ANTIMUSCARINIC AGENTS

Reference 1

39. **The tissues most sensitive to the action of Atropine are :** 103
    a) Heart
    b) Smooth muscles
    c) Skeletal muscles
    d) Salivary and Sweat glands
40. **The effect of Scopolamine on the CNS is characterised by :** 103
    a) Hallucinations
    b) Drowsiness, Amnesia and Euphoria
    c) Excitement
    d) Agitation
41. **Bradycardia caused by small doses of Atropine is due to :** Ref.2/151
    a) Stimulation of vagal center
    b) Release of acetylcholine from nerve endings
    c) Blockade of M-l receptors on postganglionic parasympathetic neurons
    d) Inhibition of the enzyme cholinesterase
42. **The effect of Atropine on the eye includes all of the following EXCEPT :** 105
    a) Passive mydriasis
    b) Cycloplegia
    c) Active mydriasis
    d) Reduction of lachrymal secretion
    e) Rise in intraocular pressure
43. **All of the following drugs selectively block M-1 receptors EXCEPT :** 105
    a) Pirenzepine
    b) Telenzepine
    c) Dicyclomine
    d) Glycopyrolate
44. **The drug which selectively blocks M-2 receptors is :** 105
    a) Trihexyphenidyl
    b) Methoctramine
    c) Dicyclomine
    d) Scopolamine
45. **The effect of Antimuscarinic agents on the gastric secretion is characterised by :** 106
    a) Blocks gastric secretion with minimum of side-effects
    b) Basal secretion is blocked more effectively than stimulated secretion

c) Stimulated secretion is blocked more effectively than basal secretion
d) More effective than Ranitidine in blocking gastric secretion

46. The drug of choice for the measurement of refractive error in young children is : 108
a) Homatropine
b) Scopolamine
c) Atropine
d) Cyclopentolate

47. The shortest acting Mydriatic-cycloplegic drug is : 108
a) Atropine
b) Homatropine
c) Cyclopentolate
d) Tropicamide

48. The Drug of choice for preventing synechia in uveitis and irritis is : 108
a) Cyclopentolate
b) Tropicamide
c) Homatropine
d) Dicyclomine

49. Antimuscarinic agent used in the treatment of bronchial asthma is : 109
a) Atropine
b) Pirenzepine
c) Ipratropium
d) Clindinium

50. The most important toxic effect produced by Atropine in infants and children is : 110
a) Hallucinations
b) Cardiac arrhythmias
c) Urinary retention
d) Hyperpyrexia
e) Convulsions

51. Cholinesterase reactivators (Oximes) are most effective in : 109
a) Blocking muscarinic effects of organophosphates
b) CNS effects of organophosphates
c) Regenerating cholinesterase at neuromuscular junction
d) Regenerating cholinesterase at all sites

52. The cholinesterase reactivator which crosses blood-brain barrier is : 109
a) Pralidoxime
b) Diacetylmonoxime
c) MINA
d) Tacrine

53. When lethal poisoning due to excessive cholinesterase inhibition is feared — as in chemical warfare — protection can be provided by pretreatment with : 110
a) Pralidoxime

b) Obodoxime
c) Pyridostigmine
d) Atropine

54. **The drug of choice for relieving bladder spasm after urologic surgery is :** 110
a) Atropine
b) Dicyclomine
c) Glycopyrrolate
d) Oxybutynin

55. **The drug of choice for treating mushroom poisoning due to A.Phalloides is :** R-2/148
a) Atropine
b) Pralidoxime
c) Ascorbic acid
d) Thioctic acid

56. **The drug of choice for the symptomatic treatment of Belladonna poisoning is :** 109
a) Neostigmine
b) Physostigmine
c) Pyridostigmine
d) DFP

ANSWERS

39.d 40.b 41.c 42.c 43.d 44.b 45.b 46.c 47.d 48.c 49.c 50.d 51.c 52.b 53.c 54.d 55.d 56.b

GANGLION BLOCKING AND NEUROMUSCULAR BLOCKING AGENTS

Reference 1

57. **The shortest acting ganglion blocking agent is :** 111
a) Atropine
b) Hexamethonium
c) Trimethaphan
d) Nicotine

58. **Trimethaphan is valuable in the treatment of all of the following EXCEPT :** 112
a) Hypertensive emergencies
b) Urinary retention
c) For producing controlled hypotension
d) Acute Pulmonary edema

59. **All of the following are long-acting skeletal muscle relaxants EXCEPT :** 408
a) Tubocurarine
b) Doxacurium
c) Metocurine
d) Atracurium

60. **The short-acting skeletal muscle relaxant is :** 408

a) Mivacurium
b) Rocuronium
c) Vecuronium
d) Pipecuronium

61. **Neuromuscular blockade may be prolonged in patients with Atypical ChE following administration of :** 409

a) Succinyl choline
b) Atracurium
c) Mivacurium
d) Drugs a and c
e) Drugs a and b

62. **The ultra-short acting skeletal muscle relaxant is :** 408

a) Mivacurium
b) Gallamine
c) Succinyl choline
d) Vecuronium

63. **The mechanism of action of nondepolarising muscle relaxants include all of the following EXCEPT :** 409

a) Competitive blockade of nicotinic receptors at NMJ
b) Blockade of the ion channels at higher doses
c) Interference with release of acetylcholine from nerve endings
d) Reduced synthesis of acetylcholine in the nerve endings

64. **Skeletal muscle relaxant with fastest onset of action is :** 412

a) Atracurium
b) Metocurine
c) Rocuronium
d) Mivacurium

65. **All of the following skeletal muscle relaxants cause hypotension EXCEPT :** 413

a) Tubocurarine
b) Atracurium
c) Mivacurium
d) Rocuronium

66. **Tachycardia induced by Pancuronium is due to :** 413

a) Vagolytic action
b) Release of noradrenaline from adrenergic nerve endings
c) Blockade of neuronal uptake of noradrenaline
d) All of the above

67. **Most common postoperative complaint of the patients receiving succinyl choline is :** 413

a) Urinary retention
b) Feeling of dizziness
c) Muscle pain
d) Nausea

68. **Neuromuscular blocking effect of nondepolarising muscle relaxants is augmented by all of the following EXCEPT :** R-2/187

a) Isoflurane
b) Aminoglycosidal antibiotics
c) Tetracyclines
d) Enflurane
e) Polymixin B
f) Erythromycin
g) Clindamycin

69. **Malignant hyperthermia following the use of inhalation anesthetic and succinyl choline is due to a defect in the :** R-2/188

a) Nicotinic receptor
b) Ryanodine receptor
c) Muscarinic receptor
d) Release of transmitter from the nerve endings

70. **Assessement of neuromuscular block is usually performed by the stimulation of :** R-2190

a) Radial nerve
b) Sciatic nerve
c) Ulnar nerve
d) Popliteal nerve

71. **The mechanism of the spasmolytic effect of Baclofen is :** 416

a) It prevents the action of acetyl choline at the NMJ
b) It prevents the destruction of GABA
c) It is an agonist at $GABA_A$ receptors
d) It is an agonist at $GABA_B$ receptors
e) All of the above

72. **The drug which reduces muscle strength by interfering with the release of calcium from the sarcoplasmic reticulum is :** 417

a) Progabide
b) Dantrolene
c) Baclofen
d) Idrocilamide
e) Glycine

73. **The skeletal muscle relaxant inactivated by Hofmann elimination is :** 408

a) Vecuronium
b) Mevacurium
c) Atracurium
d) Doxacurium

ANSWERS

57.c 58.b 59.d 60.c 61.d 62.c 63d 64.c 65.d 66.d 67.c 68.f 69.b 70.c 71.d 72.b 73.c

SYMPATHOMIMETIC AGENTS

Reference 1

74. **The drug used for the identification of the subtypes of Alpha-l receptors is :** 116
   a) Yohimbine
   b) Chloroethylclonidine
   c) Clozapine
   d) Oxymetazoline

75. **The molecular mechanism involved in mediating the responses to catecholamines is :** 117
   a) Activation of stimulatory G proteins
   b) Activation of inhibitory G proteins
   c) Activation of phospholipase C
   d) Opening of receptor-operated calcium channels
   e) All of the above

76. **The mechanism involved in desensitization of receptors, after repeated exposure to catecholamines is :** 119
   a) Receptor sequestration
   b) Down-regulation
   c) Receptor phosphorylation
   d) All of the above

77. **Catecholamines include all of the following EXCEPT :** R-2/202
   a) Adrenaline
   b) Terbutaline
   c) Isoprenaline
   d) Dopamine
   e) Colterol

78. **Pupillary dilatation caused by the sympathometics is due the activation of :** 121
   a) Alpha-2 receptors
   b) Beta-l receptors
   c) Alpha-l receptors
   d) Beta-2 receptors

79. **Activation of Alpha-2 receptors results in all of the following EXCEPT :** 121
   a) Platelet aggregation
   b) Inhibition of lipolysis
   c) Inhibition of transmitter release
   d) Glycogenolysis

80. **Selective dilatation of renal blood vessels is due to activation of :** 121
   a) Dopamine-2 receptors
   b) Beta-2 receptors
   c) Alpha-l receptors
   d) Beta-3 receptors
   e) None of the above

81. **Activation of Beta-3 receptors results in :** 121
a) Tachycardia
b) Lipolysis
c) Bronchodilatation
d) Uterine relaxation

82. **Cardiac effects of catecholamines include all of the following EXCEPT :** 122
a) Increased pacemaker activity in normal and abnormal foci
b) Increased force of contraction
c) Increased conduction velocity in A-V node
d) Improved cardiac efficiency
e) Decreased duration of systole

83. **The drug which causes mydriasis and fall in intraocular tension is :** 122
a) Atropine
b) Cyclopentolate
c) Timolol
d) Phenylephrine
e) Terbutaline

84. **Metabolic effects of catecholamines include all of the following EXCEPT :** 124
a) Increased lipolysis
b) Glycogenolysis
c) Hyperkalemia
d) Metabolic acidosis

85. **Orally active selective renal vasodilator drug is :** 125
a) Dopamine
b) Ephedrine
c) Amphetamine
d) Ibopamine

86. **The drug of choice in cardiogenic shock is :** 125
a) Dobutamine
b) Methoxamine
c) Noradrenaline
d) Dopamine

87. **The drug used to lower intraocular tension after LASER surgery is :** 129
a) Phenylephrine
b) Apraclonidine
c) Dipivefrin
d) Epinephrine
e) Timolol

88. **The drug of choice for causing uterine relaxation is :** 129
a) Salbutamol
b) Terbutaline
c) Ritodrine
d) Isoxsuprine
e) Isoetharine

89. **Therapeutic indications of Clonidine include all of the following EXCEPT :** 129

a) Hypertension

b) Treatment of diarrhea in diabetic neuropathy

c) Management of drug withdrawal

d) Treatment of rebound hypertension

e) To diminish menopausal hot flushes

90. **The sympathomimetic drug used for the treatment of Hyperkalemic familial periodic paralysis is :** R-2/208

a) Ephedrine

b) Albuterol

c) Phenylephrine

d) Salbutamol

91. **Therapeutic uses of Epinephrine include all of the following EXCEPT :** R-2/209

a) Anaphylactic shock

b) Rclief of hypersensitivity reactions

c) To reverse the effect of nonselective beta-blocking agents

d) Along with local anesthetics

92. **Catecholamine, which is a poor substrate for Monoamine oxidase, is :** R-2/212

a) Isoprenaline

b) Terbutaline

c) Dopamine

d) Noradrenaline

93. **Beta-2 selective adrenergic receptor agonist with quick onset and long duration of action is :** R-2/215

a) Terbutaline

b) Salbutamol

c) Albuterol

d) Formoterol

e) Salmeterol

ANSWERS

74.b 75.e 76.d 77.b 78.c 79.d 80.e 81.b 82.d 83.d 84.c 85.d 86.a 87.b 88.c 89.d 90.b 91.c 92.a 93.d

ADRENOCEPTOR BLOCKING AGENTS

Reference 1

94. **Restoration of responses of tissues after alpha receptor blockade by Phenoxybenzamine is dependent on :** 132

a) Excretion of the drug by the kidney

b) Synthesis of new receptors

c) Metabolism of the drug by enzymes

d) Half-life of the drug in the body

95. **The tachycardia induced by nonselective alpha receptor blocking agents is due to :** 132

a) Direct stimulation of beta receptors in the heart

b) Release of adrenaline from the adrenal medulla

c) Reflex in nature due to postural hypotension

d) Postural hypotension and blockade of presynaptic alpha-2 receptors

96. **Relatively selective alpha-l receptor blocking agents include all of the following EXCEPT :** 134

a) Terazosin

b) Phenoxybenzamine

c) Indoramine

d) Phentolamine

97. **Alpha receptor blocking agent used for treating pulmonary hypertension in the newborn infants is :** 135

a) Tolazoline

b) Phenoxybenzamine

c) Prazosin

d) Phentolamine

98. **The longest-acting selective alpha-l receptor blocking agent is :** 135

a) Terazosin

b) Indoramine

c) Doxazosin

d) Uradipil

99. **Alpha-l receptor antagonist with a weak alpha-2 agonist and a weak beta-l antagonistic action is :** 135

a) Indoramine

b) Uradipil

c) Labetalol

d) Terazosin

100. **Drugs which are relatively more selective in blocking alpha-2 receptors include all of the following EXCEPT :** 134

a) Rauwolscine

b) Yohimbine

c) Phentolamine

d) Tolazoline

101. **The drug occasionally used to treat drug-induced priapism is :** 137

a) Phentolamine

b) Phenylephrine

c) Yohimbine

d) Papavarine

102. **Metyrosin is used as an adjuvant to therapy with phenoxybenzamine in the treatment of :** 136

a) Pheochromocytoma
b) Autonomic hyperreflexia
c) Malignant pheochromocytoma
d) Benign prostatic hypertrophy

103. **The drug of choice for the management of rebound hypertension following abrupt withdrawal of Clonidine is :** 137

a) Tolazoline
b) Prazosin
c) Phenoxybenzamine
d) Phentolamine

Reference 2

104. **Alpha-l selective blocking agent that is also a potent inhibitor of cyclic nucleotide phosphodiesterase is :** 229

a) Terazosin
b) Indoramine
c) Trimazosin
d) Prazosin

105. **Finasteride, a drug used in the treatment of benign prostatic hypertrophy, produces its effect by :** 230

a) Causing relaxation of the trigone muscle
b) Relaxation of prostatic capsule and prostatic urethra
c) Inhibiting conversion of testosterone to dihydrotestosterone
d) All of the above

106. **The drug of choice for the medical management of benign prostatic hyperplasia is :** 231

a) Terazosin
b) Prazosin
c) Phenoxybenzamine
d) Alfazosin

107. **The drug which selectively blocks dopamine induced renal vasodilatation is :** 232

a) Prazosin
b) Labetalol
c) Haloperidol
d) Indoramine

Reference 1

108. **Different beta receptor blocking agents differ from each other in :** 137

a) Lipid solubility
b) Relative selectivity for beta-1 and beta-2 receptors

c) Intrinsic sympathomimetic activity

d) Membrane stabilizing activity

e) All of the above

109. **The shortest acting beta receptor blocking agent is :** 139

a) Propranolol

b) Pindolol

c) Esmolol

d) Atenolol

110. **The longest acting beta receptor blocking agent is :** 139

a) Pindolol

b) Atenolol

c) Metoprolol

d) Nadolol

111. **Increased concentrations of VLDL and decreased concentration of HDL, following chronic therapy with beta receptor blocking agents, are less likely to occur with :** 140

a) Selective beta-1 blocking agents

b) Beta blockers possessing intrinsic sympathomimetic activity

c) Drugs having membrane stabilizing activity

d) All of the above

112. **Among the adrenoceptor blocking agents, the use of which drug as antihypertensive agent has been found to be associated with no changes in plasma lipids :** 140

a) Atenolol

b) Pindolol

c) Prazosin

d) Carteolol

113. **Beta receptor blocking agent with a class III antiarrhythmic action is :** 140

a) Propranolol

b) Timolol

c) Carteolol

d) Sotalol

114. **Selective beta-1 receptor blocking agent with partial agonistic action is :** 141

a) Atenolol

b) Betaxolol

c) Acebutalol

d) Penbutalol

115. **Short duration of action of esmolol is because :** 141

a) It is rapidly hydrolised by esterases in the erythrocytes

b) It is rapidly excreted by the kidney

c) It is rapidly oxidised by cytochrome oxidase

d) It is rapidly redistributed from the site of its action

116. **Timolol is preferred for local use in the eye because of all of the following EXCEPT :** 144

a) It has no partial agonistic activity
b) It has no local anesthetic activity
c) It is a non-selective blocking agent
d) It has long duration of action
e) It is effective both orally and on local instillation

117. **Beta receptor blockade may mask the clinical signs of developing :** 145

a) Hyperglycemia
b) Angina pectoris
c) Hyperthyroidism
d) Congestive cardiac failure

118. **Beta blockers which can be used to avoid unpleasant CNS effects are :** 144

a) Acebutalol
b) Nadaolol
c) Propanolol
d) Atenolol
e) Drugs b and d
f) Drugs a and b

Reference 2

119. **Beta receptor blocking agent which lacks an effect on plasma renin activity is :** 234

a) Atenolol
b) Nodalol
c) Pindolol
d) Cartelol
e) Labetalol

120. **Pharmacological effects of Labetalol include all of the following EXCEPT :** 237

a) Selective blockade of alpha-1 receptors
b) Selective blockade of beta-1 receptors
c) Partial agonistic activity at beta-2 receptors
d) Inhibition of neuronal uptake of noradrenaline

121. **A sodium channel blocking drug that is also a beta receptor antagonist is :** 239

a) Quinidine
b) Lignocaine
c) Propafenone
d) Procainamide

122. **Selective beta-1 receptor blocking agent used topically in the treatment of glaucoma is :** 239

a) Levobunolol

b) Timolol
c) Metaprolol
d) Butaxolol
e) Atenolol

123. **The mechanism of action of propranolol in hyperthyroidism involves :** 240
a) Blockade of release of thyroxin from the thyroid gland
b) Beta receptor blockade
c) Inhibition of conversion of T-4 to T-3
d) Beta receptor blockade and inhibition of conversion of T-4 to T-3
e) Beta receptor blockade and inhibition of release of thyroxin from the gland

ANSWERS

94.b 95.d 96.d 97.a 98.c 99.b 100.c 101.b 102.c 103.d 104.d 105.c 106.d 107.c 108.e 109.c 110.d 111.b 112.c 113.d 114.c 115.a 116.c 117.c 118.e 119.c 120.b 121.c 122.d 123.d

CHAPTER 2

CARDIOVASCULAR SYSTEM

DRUGS USED IN CONGESTIVE CARDIAC FAILURE

Reference 1

1. **A negative inotropic agent which produces its action by blocking the release of calcium from the sarcoplasmic reticulum is :** 188

a) Potassium

b) Sotalol

c) Verapamil

d) Ryanodine

e) Dantroline

2. **Positive inotropic agents are effective in all types of cardiac failure EXCEPT the one associated with :** 190

a) Coronary artery disease

b) Hypertension

c) Thyrotoxicosis

d) Myocardial infarction

3. **High filling pressure of the ventricles can be reduced by all of the following EXCEPT :** 190

a) Hydralazine

b) Salt restriction

c) Diuretics

d) Nitroglycerine

4. **The first compensatory mechanism that comes into play to maintain cardiac output in CCF is :** 191

a) Vasoconstriction

b) Tachycardia

c) Retention of salt and water

d) Increased force of contraction

5. **The sugar molecule attached at number 3 position in the nucleus of cardiac glycosides influences their :** 191

a) Ability to increase force of contraction
b) Therapeutic index
c) Maximal efficacy
d) Absorption, half-life and metabolism

6. **The cardiac glycoside which is almost completely absorbed from the gut is :** 192
a) Digoxin
b) Beta-methyldigoxin
c) Deslanoside
d) Ouabain

7. **Treatment of patients, suffering from CCF, with locally acting antibiotics can increase the oral bioavailability of :** 192
a) Digoxin
b) Digitoxin
c) Deslanoside
d) Beta-methyldigoxin

8. **The cardiac glycoside which can be safely used in patients with rapidly failing renal function is :** 192
a) Digoxin
b) Beta-methyldigoxin
c) Digitoxin
d) Lanotoside-C

9. **The endogenous cardiac glycoside synthesised by adrenal medulla and released as endocrine agent, under certain circumstances like heart failure, is :** 193
a) Digoxin
b) Digitoxin
c) Bufotoxin
d) Ouabain
e) Deslanoside

10. **The positive inotropic action of cardiac glycosides is due to :** 192
a) Increase in the free calcium concentration in the vicinity of contractile protein
b) Increase of intracellular sodium concentration
c) Reduction of calcium expulsion from the cell
d) Facilitation of calcium entry through voltage-gated channels
e) All of the above
f) Mechanisms a and c

11. **The characteristics of the increase in force of contraction caused by therapeutic concentrations of cardiac glycosides include all of the following EXCEPT :** 193
a) Increased rate of development of tension
b) Prolongation of the duration of systole
c) Increased rate of relaxation
d) Little or no change in time to peak tension

12. **Digoxin increases the automaticity of all parts of the myocardium EXCEPT:**
a) Atria

b) A-V node
c) S-A node
d) Purkinje fibers

13. **Cardioselective parasympathomimetic effects produced by low doses of cardiac glycosides are due to all of the following EXCEPT :** 194
a) Sensitization of baroreceptors
b) Central vagal stimulation
c) Facilitation of muscarinic transmission at cardiac muscle
d) Release of acetylcholine from nerve endings

14. **The toxicity of cardiac glycosides is increased by all of the following EXCEPT :** 195
a) Hypokalemia
b) Hypercalcemia
c) Hypocalcemia
d) Hypomagnesemia

15. **Pharmacological effects of Milrinone include all of the following EXCEPT :** 196
a) Increased inward calcium flux
b) Selective inhibition of phosphodiesterase isoenzyme III
c) Selective inhibition of phosphodiesterase isoenzyme IV
d) Increased force of contraction
e) Vasodilatation

16. **When given at a constant dosing rate,the time required for reaching a steady state concentration with digoxin is :** 198
a) 2-3 weeks
b) 3-4 days
c) 8-10 days
d) 7 days

17. **Digitalis toxicity can be treated by all of the following EXCEPT :** 199
a) Potassium
b) Phenytoin
c) Lidocaine
d) Propranolol
e) Cardioversion

Reference 2

18. **Serum levels of digoxin required to attain maximum positive inotropic effect with minimum of toxicity are :** 815
a) 2-4 ng/ml
b) 1-1.4 ng/ml
c) 1.6-2.4. ng/ml
d) 0.5-0.75 ng/ml

19. **Absorption of digoxin is increased from the GIT by all of the following drugs EXCEPT :** 816
a) Erythromycin

b) Omeprazole
c) Tetracyclines
d) Neomycin

20. **The therapy of choice for treating life-threatening digoxin toxicity is :** 820
a) I.V. Potassium chloride
b) I.V. Lidocaine
c) Antidigoxin Fab therapy
d) I.V. Phenytoin

21. **The loop diuretic of choice for treating patients who are allergic to sulfonamides is :** 821
a) Ethacrynic acid
b) Furosemide
c) Bumetamide
d) Torsemide

22. **The only class of drugs employed in the therapy of CCF that have been shown to reduce mortality in this syndrome is :** 824
a) Cardiac glycosides
b) Diuretics
c) Beta-agonists
d) ACE inhibitors

23. **The vasodilator drug that is particularly effective in patients with CCF due to mitral regurgitation is :** 827
a) Hydralazine
b) Milrinone
c) Sodium nitroprusside
d) Minoxidil

24. **The drug which selectively inhibits platelet aggregation by inhibiting phosphodiesterase isoenzyme V is :** 833
a) Zanpiinast
b) Milrinone
c) Rolipram
d) Vinpocetine

25. **The drug which selectively inhibits phosphodiesterase isoenzyme IV and causes bronchodilatation is :** 833
a) Zanprinast
b) Aminophylline
c) Rolipram
d) Pimobendan

26. **All of the following drugs cause a positive inotropic effect and vasodilatation by inhibiting phosphodiesterase isoenzyme III EXCEPT :** 833
a) Milirinone
b) Cilostamide
c) Enoximone
d) Vesnarinone
e) Vinpocetine

ANSWERS

1.d 2.c 3.a 4.b 5.d 6.b 7.a 8.c 9.d 10.e 11.b 12.c 13.d 14.c 15.c 16.d 17.e 18.b 19.d 20.c 21.a 22.d 23.c 24.a 25.c 26.e

ANTI-ARRHYTHMIC DRUGS

Reference 1

27. **Important consequences of the reduction in peak sodium permeability and less negative resting potential include all of the following EXCEPT :** 208
    a) Reduced upstroke velocity
    b) Reduced amplitude of action potential
    c) Increased conduction velocity
    d) Reduced excitability
    e) Increase in effective refractive period

28. **The normal electrical activity in the S-A and A-V node depends on :** 210
    a) Sodium current
    b) Calcium inward current
    c) Outward potassium current
    d) Inward sodium and outward potassium current

29. **The rate of the pacemaker activity can be slowed by all of the following mechanisms EXCEPT :** 210
    a) More negative maximum diastolic potential
    b) More positive threshold potential
    c) Prolongation of the action potential duration
    d) Increase in the slope of diastolic depolarization

30. **Acceleration of the pacemaker discharge can be brought about by increase in the slope of phase 4 depolarisation caused by all of the following EXCEPT :** 211
    a) Beta receptor blockade
    b) Hypokalemia
    c) Fiber stretch
    d) Acidosis
    e) Partial depolarisation by currents of injury

31. **Match the classes given in column A with the mechanisms given in column B, as regards classification of anti-arrhythmic drugs :** 214

Column A	Column B
1. Class I	a) Calcium channel blockers
2. Class II	b) Prolongation of effective refractory period
3. Class III	c) Sodium channel blockers
4. Class IV	d) None of these
5. Class V	e) Reduced adrenergic activity

32. **Hypotension caused by I.V. Procainamide is due to :** 216

a) Alpha adrenergic blockade
b) Ganglionic blockade
c) Direct vasodilatation
d) Activation of beta receptors

33. **The anti-arrhythmic drug with minimum antimuscarinic effect is :** 215-218

a) Procainamide
b) Quinidine
c) Disopyramide
d) Imipramine

34. **Lupus erythematosus like syndrome can be caused by which of the following anti-arrhythmic drug :** 216

a) Quinidine
b) Amiodarone
c) Tocainide
d) Procainamide

35. **Anti-arrhythmic action of Amiodarone is due to :** 219

a) Blockade of sodium channels
b) Blockade of potassium channels
c) Beta adrenoceptor blockade
d) Blockade of calcium channels
e) All of the above
f) Mechanisms a and d

36. **Drugs having both anti-arrhythmic and anti-anginal effects include all of the following EXCEPT :** 219

a) Amiodarone
b) Sotalol
c) Verapamil
d) Bretyllium

37. **The therapeutic plasma concentration of Quinidine is :** 215 (in micrograms/ml)

a) 10 -15
b) 3 - 5
c) 1 - 2
d) 8 - 10

38. **Anti-arrhythmic drug that can cause fatal pulmonary fibrosis is :** 219

a) Quinidine
b) Amiodarone
c) Mexilitine
d) Phenytoin
e) Flecainide

39. **Anti-arrhythmic drug least likely to cause Torsae de pointes is :** 219

a) Quinidine
b) Bretyllium

c) Sotalol
d) Amiodarone

40. **The least cardiotoxic of the currently used antiarrhythmic drug is :** 220
a) Amiodarone
b) Lidocaine
c) Quinidine
d) Sotalol

41. **Therapeutic plasma levels of Lidocaine are (in micrograms/ml) :** 221
a) 1 - 2
b) 8 - 10
c) 2 - 6
d) 0.5 - 1

42. **24 to 36 hours may be required for attainment of steady state concentration with lidocaine in patients with :** 221
a) Liver disease
b) Kidney disease
c) Heart failure
d) Myocardial infarction

43. **Photodermatitis can be caused by which of the following antiarrhythmic drug :** 219
a) Quinidine
b) Lidocaine
c) Disopyramide
d) Amiodarone

44. **The anti-arrhythmic drug which can relieve pain due to diabetic neuropathy is :** 221
a) Phenytoin
b) Mexilitine
c) Flecainide
d) Tocainide

45. **The longest-acting anti-arrhythmic drug is :** 219
a) Mexilitine
b) Phenytoin
c) Amiodarone
d) Tocainide

46. **The shortest-acting anti-arrhythmic drug is :** 217
a) Esmolol
b) Lidocaine
c) Bretyllium
d) Adenosine

47. **The drug used primarily for the management of intraoperative arrhythmias is :** 222
a) Lidocaine

b) Esmolol
c) Adenosine
d) Bretyllium

48. **Anti-arrhythmic drug with some positive inotropic action is :** 223
a) Lidocaine
b) Quinidine
c) Bretyllium
d) Moricizine

49. **All of the following calcium channel blockers have anti-arrhythmic action EXCEPT :** 223
a) Verapamil
b) Nifedipine
c) Diltiazem
d) Bepridil

ANSWERS

27.c 28.b 29.d 30.a 31.1=c, 2=e, 3=b, 4=a 5=d 32.b 33.a 34.d 35.e 36.d 37.b 38.b 39.b 40.b 41.c 42.c 43.d 44.b 45.c 46.d 47.b 48.c 49.b

ANTI-ANGINAL DRUGS

Reference 1

50. **Regarding anti-anginal drugs all of the statements given below are correct EXCEPT :** 171
a) Some drugs act by increasing delivery of oxygen
b) All vasodilators are effective in relieving angina
c) Drugs may act by decreasing oxygen demand
d) Some agents useful in angina are not vasodilators

51. **Drugs effective in angina act by which of the following mechanisms :** 172
a) Decreasing peripheral vascular resistance
b) Decreasing cardiac output
c) Redistribution of coronary blood flow
d) Relieving coronary arterial spasm
e) All of the above

52. **The organic nitrate which has a 100% oral bioavailability is :** 173
a) Nitroglycerine
b) Isosorbide dinitrate
c) Isosorbide mononitrate
d) Pentaerythritol tetranitrate

53. **The nitrate derivative which combines the activity of NO release with potassium channel opening action is :** 174
a) Glyceryl trinitrate

b) Isosorbide dinitrate
c) Isosorbide mononitrate
d) Nicorandil

54. **The nitrate compound misused as recreational drug is :** 176
a) Isosorbide dinitrate
b) Isobutyl nitrite
c) Amyl nitrite
d) Glyceryl trinitrate

55. **Methemoglobinemia induced by nitrites is treated by I.V. :** 176
a) Sodium thiocyanate
b) Hydroxycobalamine
c) Methylene blue
d) Calcium EDTA

56. **All of the following drugs exert their vasodilating effect by causing release of nitric oxide EXCEPT :** 176
a) Glyceryl trinitrate
b) Acetylcholine
c) Sodium nitroprusside
d) Minoxidil

57. **The effectiveness of I.V. nitroglycerine to reduce infarct size and mortality fo1lowing myocardial infarction is due to its :** 176
a) Ability to reduce preload
b) Ability to cause coronary vasodilatation
c) Ability to reduce ventricular size
d) Ability to decrease platelet agrregation
e) Ability to cause redistribution of blood in the myocardium

58. **Calcium channel blockers act by blocking entry of calcium through :** 178
a) T-type channels
b) L-type channels
c) P-type channels
d) N-type channels

59. **The calcium channel blocker which is particularly effective in dilating cerebral blood vessels is :** 179
a) Amlodipine
b) Nicardipine
c) Nimodipine
d) Felodipine

60. **The calcium channel blocker which has significant sodium channel and potassium channel blocking action is :** 180
a) Verapamil
b) Diltiazem
c) Nifedipine
d) Bepridil

61. **Calcium channel blocker which has been shown to reverse the resistance of cancer cells to chemotherapeutic agents is :** 181

a) Verapamil
b) Diltiazem
c) Bepridil
d) Nicardipine

Reference 2

62. **The organic nitrate which occurs as volatile oily liquid is :** 762

a) Isosorbide dinitrate
b) Pentaerythritol tetranitrate
c) Glyceryl trinitrate
d) Erythrityl tetranitrate

63. **The relaxant effect of nitrates is somewhat unpredictable on the :** 764

a) Bronchial smooth muscle
b) Biliary tract
c) Uterine smooth muscle
d) Gastrointestinal tract

64. **The fastest velocity of metabolism of clinically used nitrate by glutathion reductase is of :** 764

a) Erythrityl tetranitrate
b) Glyceryl tetranitrate
c) Isosorbide dinitrate
d) Pentaerythritol tetranitrate

65. **The most effective approach to reduce the incidence of tolerance to nitrates during chronic therapy is :** 765

a) Prevent volume expansion with diuretics
b) Interrupt therapy for 8-12 hours each day
c) Prevent reflex neurohumoral activation
d) Combine them with sufhydril group donors

66. **All of the following are common side-effects of nitrate therapy EXCEPT :** 765

a) Headache
b) Dizziness
c) Raised intraocular pressure
d) Postural hypotension
e) Drug rash

67. **Drug rash appears to occur more commonly with :** 765

a) Nitroglycerine
b) Pentaerythritol tetranitrate
c) Isosorbide dinitrate
d) Erithrityl tetranitrate

68. **Ability of verapamil to slow A-V conduction is because :** 770

a) It reduces the magnitude of calcium current through slow channel
b) It also increases the infiuence of vagus on A-V node

c) It blocks slow calcium channels and also decreases its rate of recovery
d) In addition to blocking calcium channels it has an antiadrenergic action

69. **The calcium channel blocker which can be used in patients with A-V block or combined with beta adrenoceptor blocking agents is :** 771
a) Isradipine
b) Verapamil
c) Diltiazem
d) Nifedipine

70. **Antianginal drug which exerts some cytoprotective effects on myocardial energy metabolism is :** 776
a) Molsidamine
b) Nisoldipine
c) Flunazerine
d) Pinacidil

71. **The angiogenic factor which is being evaluated therapeutically for the treatment of angina pectoris is :** 776
a) Molsidamine
b) CGSF
c) Ranolazine
d) VEGF

ANSWERS

50.b 51.e 52.c 53.d 54.b 55.c 56.d 57.d 58.b 59.c 60.d 61.a 62.c 63.c 64.a 65.b 66.c 67.b 68.c 69.a 70.c 71.d

ANTIHYPERTENSIVE DRUGS

Reference 1

72. **The drug which possesses both diuretic and vasodilator property is :** 150
a) Chlorothiazide
b) Chlorthalidone
c) Amiloride
d) Indapamide

73. **The most common adverse effect of diuretic therapy is :** 151
a) Hypomagnessemia
b) Hypokalemia
c) Muscle weakness
d) Hyperuricemia

74. **Drugs reducing blood pressure by acting on the CNS are less likely to cause :** 151
a) Sedation
b) Nightmares

c) Postural hypotension

d) Mental depression

75. **The drug which lowers blood pressure mainly by increasing the sensitivity of baroreceptors is** : 152

a) Propranolol

b) Prazosin

c) Reserpine

d) Veratrum alkaloids

76. **The antihypertensive effect of methyldopa is blocked by the administration of** : 152

a) Diuretics

b) Inhibitors of dopa decarboxylase

c) Propranolol

d) Nifedipine

77. **Sympathoplegic hypotensive drugs are most effective when used concomitantly with** : 152

a) Nifedipine

b) Minoxidil

c) Hydrochlorthiazide

d) Enalapril

78. **The drug which produces hypotension by acting on central imidazoline receptors is** : 152

a) Rilmenidine

b) Methyldopa

c) Tolazoline

d) Guanadrel

79. **Bioavailability of methyldopa is low because it undergoes first pass metabolism in** : 153

a) Lung

b) Portal blood

c) Gastrointestinal tract

d) Liver

80. **All of the following are undesirable effects of methyldopa EXCEPT** : 153

a) Lassitude

b) Non-purepal lactation

c) Positive Coombs' test

d) Decreased renal vascular resistance

e) Nightmares

81. **The antihypertensive available as transdermal preparation is** : 153

a) Minoxidil

b) Clonidine

c) Terazosin

d) Atenolol

82. **The most frequent side-effect of clonidine is :** 153
a) Postural hypotension
b) Rebound hypertension
c) Dry mouth and sedation
d) Depression

83. **Antihypertensive effect of clonidine is blocked by the concomitant administration of :** 154
a) Nadolol
b) Tricyclic antidepressants
c) Minoxidil
d) Nifedipine

84. **Intrathecal administration of clonidine produces :** 154
a) Spinal anesthesia
b) Hypotension
c) Analgesia
d) Marked sedation

85. **Inhibition of noradrenaline release caused by Guanethidine is probably due to its :** 155
a) Local anesthetic action
b) Ability to block Uptake I
c) Analgesic action
d) Ability to deplete noradrenaline

86. **Antihypertensive effect of Guanethidine is blocked by all of the following EXCEPT :** 155
a) Cocaine
b) Amphetamine
c) Imipramine
d) Phenothiazines
e) Furosemide

87. **With regular daily dosing the onset of sympathoplegia after guanethidine occurs is about :** 156
a) 1 - 2 weeks
b) 3 - 4 days
c) 5 - 7 days
d) 3 - 4 weeks

88. **In patients taking Guanethidine-severe hypertension may result by the administration of over-the-counter preparations containing :** 156
a) Paracetamol
b) Chlorphenaramine
c) Phenylpropanolamine
d) Doxylamine

89. **The drug which acts as antihypertensive agent by formation of a false transmitter OCTOPAMINE is :** 157
a) Methyldopa

b) Pargyline
c) Reserpine
d) Clonidine

90. **In severe hypertension Propranolol is often combined with direct acting vasodilators to block beta adrenoceptors in the :** 157
a) Brain
b) GIT
c) Blood vessels
d) Heart

91. **All of the following beta-receptor blocking agents are excreted through the urine EXCEPT :** 158
a) Nadolol
b) Carteolol
c) Atenolol
d) Metoprolol
e) Betaxolol

92. **All of the following vasodilators relax arterioles EXCEPT, which relaxes both veins and arterioles :** 159
a) Minoxidil
b) Sodium nitroprusside
c) Hydralazine
d) Diazoxide

93. **The antihypertensive drug which acts through the opening of potassium channels is :** 161
a) Indoramine
b) Urapidil
c) Minoxidil
d) Pinacidil

94. **The metabolism of which of the following antihypertensive drug is bimodally distributed in the population :** 160
a) Minoxidil
b) Betaxolol
c) Enlapril
d) Hydralazine

95. **In order to prevent the development of rapid tolerance to the antihypertensive action of minoxidil it must be combined with :** 161
a) Diuretics
b) Atenolol
c) Clonidine
d) Enalapril
e) Drugs a and b
f) Drugs b and d

96. **All of the following drugs cause vasodilatation by opening potassium channels EXCEPT :** 162

a) Minoxidil
b) Uradipil
c) Cromakalin
d) Diazoxide

97. **The site of action of ACE inhibitors is** : 163
a) Liver
b) Lungs
c) Kidney
d) Brain

98. **The drug which specifically blocks angiotensin II receptors is** : 163
a) Losartan
b) Cromakalin
c) Ramipril
d) Pinacidil

99. **The drug of choice for the treatment of hypertension in diabetic patients is** : 164
a) Chlorthalidone
b) Lisinopril
c) Nadolol
d) Amlodipine

100. **All of the following ACE inhibitors are primarily eliminated by the kidney EXCEPT** : 165
a) Enlapril
b) Benzapril
c) Fosinopril
d) Quinapril
e) Ramipril

101. **Nonsteroidal anti-inflammatory agents block the hypotensive effect of ACE inhibitors by** : 165
a) Causing retention of salt and water
b) Blocking bradykinin mediated vasodilatation
c) Inhibiting the vasodilator effect of ACE inhibitors
d) Causing vasoconstriction

102. **The commonest side-effect — cough — of ACE inhibitors is due to** : 165
a) Irritation of bronchi
b) Stimulation of cough center
c) Production of bradykinin and prostaglandins
d) Irritation of GIT

Reference 2

103. **When used as monotherapy, the maximal daily dose of thiazide (Hydrochlorthiazide) diuretics should not exceed** : 782
a) 50 mg/day
b) 25 mg/day

c) 100 mg/day

d) 75 mg/day

104. **Attenuation of the kaliuretic effect of thiazide diuretics can be achieved by combining them with all of the following EXCEPT :** 783

a) Amiloride

b) Enalapril

c) Acetazolamide

d) Spironolactone

105. **The antihypertensive effect of all thiazide diuretics is progressively diminished when the GFR falls below 30 ml/mt EXCEPT :** 783

a) Hydrochlorthiazide

b) Benzthiazide

c) Metolazone

d) Indapamide

106. **Surrogate markers used to evaluate effectiveness of long term therapy with diuretics include all of the following EXCEPT :** 783-4

a) Systolic B.P.

b) Hypokalemia

c) Glycoselated hemoglobin

d) LDL levels

e) Hyperuricemia

107. **Most effective diuretic, as antihypertensive agent, in patients with normal renal function are :** 785

a) Carbonic anhydrase inhibitors

b) Loop diuretics

c) Thiazide diuretics

d) Potassium sparing diuretics

108. **The potassium retaining effect of potassium sparing diuretics can be increased by all of the following, resulting in hyperkalemia, EXCEPT :** 786

a) Propranolol

b) Minoxidil

c) Enalapril

d) Ibuprofen

109. **Loss of therapeutic effect following high doses of Clonidine and Guanfacine is due to :** 788

a) Inability of high doses to cross blood-brain barrier

b) Release of noradrenaline from adrenergic nerve endings

c) Tachycardia and increased cardiac output

d) Activation of alpha-2 receptors on vascular smooth muscle

e) None of the above

110. **The alpha-2 adrenergic agonist which can cause water diuresis due to inhibition of release and renal actions of vasopressin is :** 789

a) Guanbenz

b) Clonidine

c) Guanfacine
d) Noradrenaline

111. **Parotid gland swelling and pain is caused by which of the following antihypertensive agent :** 789

a) Hydrochlorthiazide
b) Hydralazine
c) Methyldopa
d) Clonidine

112. **The antihypertensive agent which is more likely to cause severe hypertension if used during the withdrawal syndrome following discontinuation of alpha-2 adrenergic agonist is :** 789

a) Spironolactone
b) Alpha methyldopa
c) Hydralazine
d) Propranolol
e) Labetalol

113. **Secretion of renin is reduced by all of the following antihypertensive agents EXCEPT :** 787, 88, 90, 92

a) Alpha methyldopa
b) Clonidine
c) Guanethidine
d) Propranolol
e) Enalapril

114. **The antihypertensive agent that can be labelled as a fixed-dose combination of two drugs is :** 794

a) Enalapril
b) Atenolol
c) Labetalol
d) Dilevalol

115. **Paradoxical hypertensive reactions to beta adrenoceptor blocking agents can occur under which of the following situations :** 793

a) Hypoglycemia
b) In patients with pheochromocytoma
c) During withdrawal from clonidine
d) Administration of epinephrine
e) All of the above

116. **Pyridoxine responsive polyneuropathy is caused by which of the following agents :** 795

a) Minoxidil
b) Hydralazine
c) Labetalol
d) Enalapril

117. **In case of hydralazine, the rate of acetylation is an important determinant of :** 795

a) Bioavailability
b) Degree of elimination
c) Duration of action
d) Degree of tachycardia produced

118. **The antihypertensive drug which is inactive in causing relaxation of smooth muscle in vitro is :** 796
a) Nifedipine
b) Diazoxide
c) Minoxidil
d) Sodium nitroprusside

119. **All of the following vasodilators cause an overall increase in myocardial oxygen demand EXCEPT :** 798
a) Hydralazine
b) Sodium nitroprusside
c) Minoxidil
d) Diazoxide

120. **Rebound hypertension can occur following abrupt cessation of therapy with all of the following drugs EXCEPT :** 798
a) Sodium nitroprusside
b) Beta adrenoceptor blocking agents
c) Clonidine
d) Minoxidil

121. **Hyperglycemia caused by Diazoxide is due to :** 801
a) Increased absorption of glucose from GIT
b) Glycogenolysis
c) Neoglucogenesis
d) Inhibition of release of insulin from pancreas
e) None of the above

122. **Edema caused by Calcium channel blockers is due to :** 801
a) Retention of salt and water
b) Increased hydrostatic pressure following precapillary dilatation
c) Decreased renal blood flow
d) Reduced osmotic pressure

123. **The probable mechanism by which obesity causes hypertension is :** 804
a) Increased absorption of fat from GIT
b) Increased secretion of insulin with retention of salt and water
c) Retention of vasoconstrictor substances
d) Inhibition of lipolysis

124. **The mechanism by which Angiotensin II increases total peripheral resistance is :** 740-741
a) Direct vasoconstriction
b) Enhancement of peripheral noradrenergic transmission
c) Increased sympathetic discharge from CNS

d) Release of catecholamines from adrenal medulla
e) All of the above
f) Mechanisms a and d

125. **All of the following ACE inhibitors are PRODRUGS EXCEPT** : 745-46
a) Enalapril
b) Lisinopril
c) Benazepril
d) Fosinopril
e) Spirapril

126. **Which of the group of drugs augment the antihypertensive response to ACE inhibitors by rendering the patient's B.P. renin-dependent** : 747
a) Calcium channel blockers
b) Alpha adrenergic receptor blockers
c) Diuretics
d) Beta adrenoceptor blocking agents

127. **Which of the following antihypertensive agent can cause DYSGEUSIA in some patients** : 751
a) Caclium channel blockers
b) Beta adrenoceptor blocking agents
c) Diuretics
d) Adrenergic neurone blocking agents
e) ACE inhibitors

128. **The antihypertensive agent, acting through renin-angiotensin system, which induces a significant uricosuric effect is** : 753
a) Enalapril
b) Fosinopril
c) Losartan
d) Spirapril
e) Benazapril

ANSWERS

72.d 73.b 74.c 75.d 76.b 77.c 78.a 79.c 80.d 81.b 82c 83.b 84.c 85.a 86.e 87.a 88.c 89.b 90.d 91.e 92.b 93.c 94.d 95.e 96.b 97.b 98.a 99.b 100.c 101.b 102.c 103b 104.c 105.c 106.e 107.c 108.b 109.d 110.a 111.d 112.d 113.c 114.c 115.e 116.b 117.a 118.c 119.b 120.d 121.d 122.b 123.b 124.e 125.b 126.c 127.e 128.c

CHAPTER 3

DIURETICS

Reference 1

1. **The only diuretic which acts on the proximal tubule is :** 230
   a) Osmotic diuretics
   b) Spironolactone
   c) Acetazolamide
   d) Chlorothiazide

2. **Metabolic acidosis produced by carbonic anhydrase inhibitors may be responsible for their effectiveness in all of the following conditions EXCEPT :** R-2/695
   a) Epilepsy
   b) Acute mountain sickness
   c) Familiar periodic paralysis
   d) Glaucoma

3. **Pharmacological effects of loop diuretics include all of the following EXCEPT :** 237-38
   a) Inhibition of NaCl absorption in the thick ascending limb of loop of Henele
   b) Increased magnesium and calcium excretion
   c) Their diuresis is limited by the development of acidosis
   d) Redistribution of renal blood flow within the cortex

4. **Indications of loop diuretics include all of the following EXCEPT :** 238
   a) Acute pulmonary edema
   b) Hyperkalemia
   c) Acute renal failure
   d) Hypercalciuria
   e) Anion overdose

5. **The thiazide diuretic which is primarily excreted by the biliary system is :** 239
   a) Indapamide
   b) Chlorothiazide
   c) Polythiazide
   d) Benzthiazide

6. Hyperglycemia induced by thiazide diuretics is due to : 240

a) Glycogenolysis
b) Neoglucogenesis
c) Impaired release of insulin and diminished utilisation of glucose
d) Increased absorption of glucose

7. The combination of which of the following diuretic with Indomethacin has been reported to cause Acute Renal failure : 242

a) Triamterene
b) Spironolactone
c) Hydrochlorthiazide
d) Amiloride

8. Lithium induced polyuria can be partially reversed by : 247

a) Hydrochlorthiazide
b) Amiloride
c) Furosemide
d) Mannitol

Reference 2

9. All of the following drugs inhibit carbonic anhydrase found in luminal and basolateral membrane (type IV) as well as in the cytoplasm (type II) EXCEPT : 691

a) Acetazolamide
b) Benzolamide
c) Dichlorphenamide
d) Methazolamide

10. The mechanism of "diuretic braking" involves : 691

a) Activation of renin angiotensin system
b) Decreased arterial pressure
c) Hypertrophy of the renal epithelial cells
d) Increased expression of renal epithelial transporters
e) Mechanism a and d
f) All of the above

11. The primary site of action of osmotic diuretics is : 696

a) Loop of Henele
b) Proximal convoluted tubule
c) Collecting ducts
d) Distal convoluted tubule
e) All of the above

12. The loop diuretic which is a sulfonyl urea derivative is : 697

a) Furosemide
b) Torsemide
c) Azosemide
d) Piretenide

13. The loop diuretic which is particularly effective in reducing left ventricular pressure is : 700

a) Ethacrynic acid
b) Torsemide
c) Furosemide
d) Azosemide

14. **The loop diuretic which is likely to induce ototoxicity more often than other agents is :** 700
a) Furosemide
b) Torsemide
c) Piretinide
d) Ethacrynic acid

15. **The longest acting thiazide-like diuretic is :** 703
a) Indapamide
b) Chlorthalidone
c) Polythiazide
d) Hydroflumethiazide

16. **The effect of loop and thiazide diuretics on uric acid excretion is :** 699-722
a) Excretion is decreased
b) Excretion is increased
c) No effect on excretion
d) Acute administration increases while chronic administration decreases excretion

17. **Thiazide diuretics diminish the effect of all of the following EXCEPT :** 704
a) Anticoagulants
b) Uricosuric agents
c) Diazoxide
d) Sulfonylureas

18. **Which of the following diuretics can cause megaloblastic anemia :** 706
a) Amiloride
b) Triamterine
c) Spironolactone
d) Furosemide

19. **The diuretic which has been shown to improve mucociliary clearance in patients with cystic fibrosis is :** 706
a) Amiloride
b) Triamterine
c) Acetazolamide
d) Muzolimine

ANSWERS

1.c 2.d 3.c 4.d 5.a 6.c 7.a 8.b 9.b 10.f 11.a 12.b 13.c 14.d 15.b 16.d 17.c 18.b 19.a

CHAPTER 4

HISTAMINE AND ANTIHISTAMINICS

Reference 1

1. **All of the following amines are metabolised by MAO EXCEPT : 251**
   a) Noradrenaline
   b) Histamine
   c) Dopamine
   d) Serotonine
   e) Tyramine
2. **Histamine-3 receptors are located presynaptically in the : 253**
   a) Smooth muscles
   b) Gastric mucosa
   c) Brain and Myentric plexus
   d) Cardiac muscles
3. **Activation of H_3 receptors results in the reduction of release of all of the following transmitters EXCEPT : 252**
   a) Histamine
   b) Serotonin
   c) Norepinephrine
   d) Acetylcholine
   e) Dopamine
4. **All of the following effects are due to the activation of H_1 receptors EXCEPT : 253-4**
   a) Edema
   b) Cardiovascular responses
   c) Bronchoconstriction
   d) Pain and itching
   e) Contraction of smooth muscles
5. **The drug which is an agonist at H_2 receptors and antagonist at H_3 receptors is : 254**
   a) Triplolidine

b) Thiperamine
c) Tiotidine
d) Impromodine

6. **The drug which is a potent and selective H_3 receptor agonist is :** 254
a) 2-Methyl histamine
b) R-alpha methyl histamine
c) 4-methyl histamine
d) Betazole

7. **The selective antagonist for H_3 receptors is :** 255
a) Thioperamide
b) Impromidine
c) Tiotidine
d) Triplolidine

8. **All of the following antihistaminics enter the CNS EXCEPT :** 256
a) Cyclizine
b) Diphenhydramine
c) Antazoline
d) Chlorpheniramine
e) Astemizole

9. **The antihistaminic which is most likely to cause postural hypotension in susceptible individuals is :** 258
a) Meclizine
b) Terfenadine
c) Promethazine
d) Pyrilamine

10. **All of the following drugs are effective in controlling motion sickness and vestibular disturbances EXCEPT :** 258
a) Scopolamine
b) Promethazine
c) Diphenhydramine
d) Cyclizine
e) Cetrizine

11. **The antihistaminic which can cause potentially lethal ventricular arrhythmias if given with Ketoconazole or Erythromycin is :** 259
a) Promethazine
b) Ranitidine
c) Terfenadine
d) Doxylamine

12. **The H_2 receptor antagonist which stimulates the contractile activity of stomach due to its ability to inhibit the enzyme cholinesterase is :** 260
a) Cimetidine
b) Ranitidine
c) Nizatidine
d) Famotidine

Reference 2

13. **The antihistaminic which is primarily excreted renally unmetabolized is :** 590
    a) Terfenadine
    b) Diphenhydramine
    c) Astemizole
    d) Cetrizine
    e) Pyrilamine
14. **Non mast cell sites of histamine formation or storage include all of the following EXCEPT :** 582
    a) Bronchial tree
    b) Epidermis
    c) Gastric mucosa
    d) Neurons in the CNS
    e) Cells in rapidly regenerating tissues
15. **All of the following effects of Histamine on the heart are mediated through H_2 receptors EXCEPT :** 585
    a) Increased force of contraction
    b) Tachycardia
    c) Slowed A-V conduction
    d) Increased automaticity

ANSWERS

1.b 2.c 3.e 4.b 5.d 6.b 7.a 8.e 9.c 10.e 11.c 12.c 13.d 14.a 15.c

CHAPTER 5

GASTRO-INTESTINAL SYSTEM

Reference 2

1. **The H_2 receptor antagonist which has little or no effect on acid secretion but can antagonize the effects of histamine in CNS is :** 904
   a) Ranitidine
   b) Nizatidine
   c) Famotidine
   d) Zolentidine

2. **Pharmacological effects of H_2 receptor antagonists include all of the following EXCEPT :** 904-5
   a) Inhibition of gastric acid secretion by histamine and other H_2 receptor agonists
   b) Inhibition of acid secretion elicited by gastrin and muscarinic agonist
   c) Inhibition of basal, nocturnal and stimulated acid secretion
   d) Reduction of both volume of gastric juice secreted and its H^+ ion concentration
   e) Antagonise the effects mediated by H_2 receptors on vascular and bronchial muscles

3. **The H_2 receptor antagonist which has maximum oral bioavailability is :** 905
   a) Nizatidine
   b) Famotidine
   c) Ranitidine
   d) Zolentidine

4. **All of the following H_2 receptor antagonists are excreted in large part in the urine without being metabolized in the liver EXCEPT :** 905
   a) Nizatidine
   b) Ranitidine
   c) Zolentitidine
   d) Famotidine

5. **Antacids decrease the bioavailability of all of the following drugs EXCEPT :** 912
   a) Iron
   b) Tetracyclines
   c) Quinolone antibiotics
   d) Isoniazide

4

e) Metoprolol
f) Theophylline

6. All of the following are congeners of PGE_2, which are under study for usefulness in the therapy of peptic ulcer EXCEPT : 914

a) Rioprostil
b) Arboprostil
c) Enprostil
d) Trimoprostil

7. The osmotic laxative which is helpful in managing chronic hepatic encephalopathy is : 922

a) Glycerine
b) Lactulose
c) Sorbitol
d) Mannitol

8. Atropine is added to diphenoxylate in antidiarrheal preparation mainly to : 926

a) Potentiate its antidiarrheal action
b) Block its cholinergic side-effects
c) Discourage abuse of this opioid preparation
d) Reduce systemic absorption of diphenoxylate

9. The drug of choice for treating idiopathic diarrhea in AIDS patients is : 928

a) Bismuth salicylate
b) Diphenoxylate
c) Difenoxin
d) Octreotide
e) Loperamide

10. The antibiotic which acts as a prokinetic agent by stimulating motilin receptors is : 932

a) Tetracycline
b) Streptomycin
c) Ciprofloxacin
d) Erythromycin
e) Rifampin

ANSWERS

1.d 2.e 3.a 4.b 5.e 6.a 7.b 8.c 9.d 10.d

CHAPTER 6

HEMOPOIETIC SYSTEM

HAEMATINICS

Reference 1

1. **The most important site of iron absorption is :** 493
   a) Stomach
   b) Duodenum
   c) Jejunum
   d) Duodenum and proximal jejunum
   e) Jejunum and proximal ileum
2. **The most important factor regulating iron absorption is :** 494
   a) Mucosal block
   b) Iron requirement of the body
   c) Dose of the iron given
   d) Preparation of the iron given
3. **Iron absorption is increased by :** 494
   a) Tetracyclines
   b) Antacids
   c) Reducing substances
   d) Phytates
4. **To raise the hemoglobin concentration of blood by 1 g/dl the amount of elemental iron required is :** 495
   a) 200 mgm
   b) 400 mgm
   c) 300 mgm
   d) 600 mgm
5. **65 mgm of elemental iron is present in :** 495
   a) 200 mgm of hydrated Ferrous sulfate
   b) 320 mgm of Ferrous gluconate
   c) 200 mgm of desiccated Ferrous sulfate
   d) 325 mgm of Ferrous .fumarate

6. **Regarding correction of iron deficiency which of the following statement is most appropriate :** 495

a) Parentral iron corrects the deficiency more rapidly

b) Sustained release preparations are more suited as they provide continuous release

c) Oral iron in the form of desiccated Ferrous sulfate is the preparation of choice

d) Oral iron corrects the deficiency just as rapidly as parenteral iron in most cases

7. **In the treatment of iron deficiency anemias,therapy with oral iron should be continued for :** 495

a) 2-3 months after the hemoglobin level returns to normal

b) 2-4 weeks after the hemoglobin level returns to normal

c) 3-6 months after the hemoglobin level returns to normal

d) 8-12 months after the hemoglobin level returns to normal

8. **Failure to respond to oral iron therapy may be due to :** 495

a) Incorrect diagnosis

b) Continued blood loss

c) Poor compliance by the patient

d) Inflammatory bowel disese

e) Statements b and c

f) All of the statements a to d

9. **Indications for parenteral iron therapy include all of the following EXCEPT :** 495

a) Inflammatory bowel disease

b) To increase the hemoglobin concentration rapidly

c) Chronic bleeding

d) Small bowel resection

e) Unreliable patient

10. **Among the parenteral iron preparations, iron dextran complex is preferred over iron sorbitol citric acid complex because :** 496

a) It acts more rapidly

b) Chances of adverse reactions are less

c) It is less irritant

d) It is easily available

e) It can be given both I.M. and I.V.

11. **The specific antidote for treating acute iron toxicity is :** 496

a) EDTA

b) Desferoxamine

c) BAL

d) Penicillamine

12. **Chronic iron overload is most effectively treated by :** 496

a) Oral desferoxamine

b) Parenteral desferoxamine

c) Intermittent phlebotomy

d) Oral DTPA

13. Which of the following chelating agents forms a toxic compound with iron and hence should not be used to treat iron toxicity : 496

a) EDTA
b) Penicillamine
c) BAL
d) DTPA

14. The active form of Vitamin B_{12} is : 497

a) Deoxyadenosylcobalamine
b) Hydroxycobalamine
c) Methylcobalamine
d) Forms a and c
e) Forms b and c

15. The main site of absorption of vitamin B_{12} after oral administration is : 498

a) Stomach
b) Duodenum
c) Proximal ileum
d) Distal ileum

16. Once absorbed, vitamin B_{12} is transported to various cells bound to : 498

a) Transcobalamin I
b) Transcobalamin III
c) Transcobalamin II
d) Intrinsic factor

17. The enzyme involved in the hydrolysis of polyglutamates present in the diet to monoglutamates is : 499

a) Methylmalonyl Co A
b) Alpha-L-glutamyl transferase
c) Succinyl coenzyme A
d) Methyltranferase

18. Metabolic functions of Folic acid include all of the following EXCEPT : 500

a) Conversion of homocysteine to methionine
b) Generation of thymidilate
c) Conversion of malonic acid to succinic acid
d) Conversion of serine to glycine
e) Generation of formate pool

19. Neurological manifestations of vitamin B_{12} deficiency are due to : 499

a) Non-conversion of homocysteine to methionine
b) Non-conversion of methylmalonyl Co A to Succinyl Co A
c) Non-conversion of serine to glycine
d) Abnormal histidine metabolism

20. Maternal deficiency of Folic acid in pregnant women may cause in the fetus : 502

a) Hair-lip
b) Spina bifida

c) Early closure of ductus arteriosus
d) Retarded growth in the fetus
e) All of the above

21. **Parenteral Hydroxycobalamine is preferred over Cyanocobalamine for treating Vit. B_{12} deficiency because :** 502
a) It is better absorbed
b) It causes less irritation at the site of injection
c) It corrects the deficiency more rapidly
d) It is highly bound to proteins, so remains longer in circulation
e) It can be given both I.M. and I.V.

22. **Megaloblastic anemia due to Folic acid deficiency can occur following the administration of all of the following drugs EXCEPT :** 502
a) Phenytoin
b) Trimethoprim
c) Pyrimethamine
d) Indomethacin
e) Oral contraceptives
f) Isoniazide

23. **Endogenous Erythropoietin is produced by :** 503
a) Liver
b) Bone marrow
c) Kidney
d) Adrenal gland

24. **The drug of choice for treating the anemia of chronic renal failure and Zidovudine- induced anemia is :** 504
a) Parenteral iron
b) Vitamin B_{12}
c) Folic acid
d) GM-CSF
e) Erythropoietin

ANSWERS

1.d 2.b 3.c 4.a 5.c 6.d 7.c 8.f 9.b 10.e 11.b 12.c 13.c 14.d 15.d 16.c 17.b 18.c 19.b 20.b 21.d 22.d 23.c 24.e

DRUGS USED IN DISORDERS OF COAGULATION

Reference 1

25. **The sequence of events occurring in immediate hemostatic response is :** 507
a) Platelet aggregation-platelet adhesion-vasospasm-viscous metamorphosis-fibrin deposition
b) Vasospasm-platelet adhesion-platelet aggregation-viscous metamorphosis-fibrin deposition

c) Platelet adhesion-vasospasm-platelet aggregation-viscous metamorphosis-fibrin deposition

d) Vasopsasm-viscous metamorphosis-fibrin deposition-platelet adhesion-platelet aggregation

26. **Regarding Thromboxane A_2 which of the following statement is most appropriate :** 507

a) It is synthesised in the vessel wall and inhibits thrombogenesis

b) It is synthesised in the platelets and inhibits thrombogenesis

c) It is synthesised in the platelets and induces thrombogenesis

d) It is synthesised in the platelets and induces thrombogenesis & vasoconstriction

27. **Regarding Prostacycline which of the following statement is most appropriate :** 507

a) It is synthesised in the platelets and inhibits thrombogenesis

b) It is synthesised in the vessel wall and inhibits thrombogenesis

c) It is synthesised in the vessel wall and induces thrombogenesis

d) It is synthesised in the platelets and induces thrombogenesis

28. **The most important mechanism of action of Heparin is :** 509

a) It promotes aggregation of platelets

b) It inhibits synthesis of prothrombin in the liver

c) It catalyses the antithrombin-protease reaction

d) It inhibits the synthesis of important clotting factors

29. **Low molecular weight heparin differs from standard heparin in all of the following respects EXCEPT :** 509

a) It has equal or greater efficacy

b) It causes lower incidence of bleeding

c) It is to be given more frequently

d) There is less need for laboratory monitoring

e) Increased bioavailability from S.C. injection site

30. **The salt of heparin used as in vitro anticoagulant is :** 509

a) Sodium heparin

b) Lithium heparin

c) Potassium heparin

d) Calcium heparin

31. **One mgm. of sodium heparin ((USP) contains :** 509

a) 140 units

b) 130 units

c) 200 units

d) 120 units

32. **Toxic effects of heparin include all of the following EXCEPT :** 509

a) Bleeding

b) Alopecia

c) Paradoxical thromboembolism

d) Osteoporosis

e) Thrombocytopenia
f) Osteomalacia

33. **Contraindications for the use of heparin include all of the following EXCEPT :** 510
a) Active bleeding
b) Hemophilia
c) Infective endocarditis
d) Purpura
e) Venous thrombosis
f) Threatened abortion

34. **The route by which heparin is never administered is :** 510
a) Intravenous
b) Subcutaneous
c) Intramuscular
d) None of these

35. **The dose of heparin is regulated by which of the following laboratory test :** 510
a) Prothrombin time
b) Bleeding time
c) Clotting time
d) Partial thromboplastin time

36. **The specific antidote for heparin is :** 511
a) Vitamin K
b) Protamin sulfate
c) EDTA
d) Blood transfusion

37. **The anticoagulant that is widely used as rodenticide is :** 511
a) Heparin
b) Dicumarol
c) Warfarin
d) Sodium sulfate

38. **The anticoagulant which is effective both orally and parenterally is :** 511
a) Heparin
b) Dicumarol
c) Phenindione
d) Warfarin

39. **The mechanism of action of oral anticoagulants is :** 512
a) They prevent platelet aggregation
b) They act as antithrombin
c) They inhibit activation of prothrombin and factors VII, IX and X
d) They inhibit release of prothrombin from liver

40. **Genetic resistance to warfarin in humans is due to :** 512
a) Deficiency of vitamin K epoxoide reductase
b) Mutational change in vitamin K epoxoide reductase

c) Excess of vitamin K epoxoide reductase

d) Presence of warfarin hydrolysases

41. **The dose of warfarin is regulated by which of the following laboratory test :** 513

a) Bleeding time

b) Partial thromboplastin time

c) Prothrombin time

d) Clotting time

42. **The anticoagulant effect of warfarin is increased by all of the following EXCEPT :** 514

a) Phenylbutazone

b) Sulfinpyrazone

c) Metronidazole

d) Miconazole

e) Indomethacin

43. **The anticoagulant effect of warfarin is decreased by all of the following EXCEPT :** 514

a) Phenobarbitone

b) Rifampin

c) Cholestyramine

d) Acetaminophen

e) Vitamin K

f) Chlorthalidone

44. **To reduce the incidence of bleeding due to non-selective effect of fibrinolytic agents, they are best administered :** 515

a) Subcutaneously

b) Intravenously

c) Orally

d) Intra-arterially

e) Per rectum

45. **Advantages of ANISTREPLASE over STREPTOKINASE include all of the following EXCEPT :** 515

a) It can be given rapidly Intravenously

b) It has greater clot selectivity

c) It can be prepared by recombinant DNA technology

d) It has more thrombolytic activity

46. **Indications for the use of fibrinolytic agents include all of the following EXCEPT :** 515

a) Pulmonary embolism

b) Venous thrombosis

c) Acute myocardial infarction

d) Peripheral vascular disease

e) None of the above

47. **Aspirin is preferred over other non-steroidal anti-inflammatory drugs for antithrombotic action because :** 516

a) It inhibits both cyclooxygenase and prostacyclin synthase enzymes
b) It is an irreversible inhibitor of cyclooxygenase enzyme
c) It is relatively non-toxic
d) It has additional analgesic-antipyretic actions

48. **The drug which reduces platelet aggregation by inhibiting ADP-induced platelet aggregation is :** 516

a) Aspirin
b) Sulfinpyrazone
c) Ticlopidine
d) Indomethacin
e) Ethanol

49. **The drug of choice for treating Hemophilia and von Willibrand's disease is :** 518

a) Vitamin K
b) Menaquinone
c) Ticlopidine
d) Cryoprecipitate
e) Aspirin

50. **All of the following drugs increase the factor VIII activity in patients with mild Hemophilia A EXCEPT :** 519

a) Cryoprecipitate
b) Phytonadione
c) Desmopressin acetate
d) Danazol

51. **The drug which inhibits fibrinolysis is :** 519

a) Danazol
b) Aspirin
c) Menadione
d) Tranexamic acid
e) Autoplex

ANSWERS

25.b 26.d 27.b 28.c 29.c 30.b 31.d 32.f 33.e 34.c 35.d 36.b 37.c 38.d 39.c 40.b 41.c 42.e 43.d 44.d 45.c 46.e 47.b 48.c 49.d 50.b 51.d

HYPOLIPIDEMIC AGENTS

52. **The condition involving increased levels of Triglycerides in the plasma is known as :** 522

a) Hyperlipidemia
b) Hyperlipoproteinemia
c) Hyperlipemia
d) Hypercholesterimia

53. **Acute pancreatitis and atherosclerosis are the two important sequelae of :** 522
 a) Hyperlipoproteinimia
 b) Hyperlipemia
 c) Diabetes mellitus with hyperlipemia
 d) Hypertension with hyperlipemia

54. **All of the following are atherogenic lipoproteins EXCEPT :** 522
 a) LDL
 b) VLDL
 c) IDL
 d) HDL
 e) Lp (a) lipoproteins

55. **The most important adjunct to drug therapy of hyperlipidemias is :** 528
 a) Exercise
 b) Avoid smoking and alcohol
 c) Diet
 d) All of the above

56. **Match the mechanism of action of drugs given in Column A with the mechanism given in Column B :** 529-33

Column A	Column B
1. Niacin	a) Reduces VLDL levels by increasing the activity of lipoprotein lipase
2. Colestepol	b) Inhibits secretion of VLDL by the liver
3. Gemfibrozil	c) Competitive inhibitor of HMG-Co A reductase
4. Probucol	d) Antioxidant. Also inhibits sterol synthesis
5. Lovastatin	e) Prevents reabsorption of bile acids from the intestinal lumen

57. **The best time for the administration of HMG-Co A reductase inhibitors is :** 532
 a) Early in the morning
 b) After lunch
 c) In the evening
 d) At bed time
 e) Can be given at any time in the day

58. **The most important toxic effect of Lovastatin is :** 533
 a) GIT upset
 b) Hyperglycemia
 c) Thrombocytopenia
 d) Neuropathy
 e) Myopathy

ANSWERS

52.c 53.a 54.d 55.c 56.1=b, 2=e, 3=a, 4=d, 5=c 57.c 58.e

CHAPTER 7

CENTRAL NERVOUS SYSTEM

GENERAL ANESTHETICS

Reference 1

1. The rate of induction of anesthesia is fastest with : 383

a) Enflurane
b) Nitrous oxide
c) Halothane
d) Isoflurane

2. The rate of recovery from anesthesia is most rapid with : 386

a) Sevoflurane
b) Isoflurane
c) Halothane
d) Desflurane

3. The rate of recovery with halothane is more rapid than that of enflurane because : 386

a) It is less soluble in blood as compared to enflurane
b) It causes hyperventilation
c) 15 to 20 % of inspired halothane is metabolised during an average anesthetic procedure
d) It increases pulmonary blood flow exposing a larger volume of blood from which anesthetic can be washed out

4. In terms of Minimum Alveolar Concentration (MAC) the most potent anesthetic is : 383

a) Nitrous oxide
b) Desflurane
c) Isoflurane
d) Enflurane
e) Halothane

5. All of the following anesthetic agents cause an increase in heart rate EXCEPT : 388

a) Methoxyflurane
b) Halothane
c) Enflurane
d) Isoflurane

6. **All of the inhaled anesthetics, in current use,cause a decrease in tidal volume and an increase in respiratory rate EXCEPT :** 388

a) Halothane
b) Desflurane
c) Isoflurane
d) Enflurane
e) Nitrous oxide

7. **All of the following anesthetics are potent uterine relaxants EXCEPT :** 389

a) Nitrous oxide
b) Halothane
c) Isoflurane
d) Enflurane

8. **Vasopressin-resistant polyuric renal insufficiency is caused by which of the following anesthetic agent :** 389

a) Halothane
b) Desflurane
c) Methoxyflurane
d) Isoflurane
e) Ketamine

9. **Prolonged exposure to which of the following anesthetic agent can cause Megaloblastic anemia :** 390

a) Ether
b) Isoflurane
c) Enflurane
d) Etomidate
e) Nitrous oxide

10. **All of the following anesthetic agents can increase intracranial pressure EXCEPT :** 388

a) Halothane
b) Isoflurane
c) Desflurane
d) Enflurane

11. **Midazolam is preferred over other benzodiazepines for use in anesthetic procedures because :** 391

a) Midazolam formulations are water-soluble
b) It has a rapid onset and shorter elimination half-life
c) It has a steeper dose response curve
d) It causes anterograde amnesia
e) All of the above
f) Statements b and d

12. **The shortest acting opioid analgesic used in anesthetic practice is :** 391

a) Morphine
b) Alfentanyl
c) Fentanyl
d) Sufentanyl

13. **The drug combination used with Nitrous oxide to provide Neuroleptanesthesia is :** 391

a) Morphine + Droperidol
b) Fentanyl + Droperidol
c) Fentanyl + Haloperidol
d) Morphine + Haloperidol

14. **Propofol is popular as anesthetic use in "day surgery" because of all of the following EXCEPT :** 391

a) It has a rapid onset of action
b) Recovery is more rapid and patient can ambulate sooner
c) It has no effect on blood pressure
d) Post operative vomiting is uncommon as it is reported to have antiemetic effect

15. **Which of the following anesthetic agent causes an effect termed "Emergence Phenomenon" during recovery :** 392

a) Diazepam
b) Midazolam
c) Propofol
d) Ketamine
e) Etomidate

Reference 2

16. **Because of the development of the concept of "Balanced anesthesia", the principal factor that now determines the acceptibility of a general anesthetic agent is :** 307

a) Rapid and pleasant induction of and recovery from anesthesia
b) Wide margin of safety
c) Incidence of adverse effects
d) Degree of relaxation of skeletal muscles
e) Rapid control in the depth of anesthesia

17. **All of the following are advantages of Halothane EXCEPT :** 313

a) It is nonflammable
b) Induction and recovery from anesthesia are not prolonged
c) It is a good analgesic
d) It is a good uterine relaxant

18. **The use of all of the following anesthetic agents has been associated with the occurrence of malignant hyperthermia EXCEPT :** 318

a) Desflurane
b) Enflurane

c) Halothane
d) Isoflurane

19. **Intravenous anesthetic agent which exists as an oil at room temperature is** : 327
a) Ketamine
b) Romifentyl
c) Etomidate
d) Propofol

ANSWERS

1.b 2.d 3.c 4.e 5.b 6.e 7.a 8.c 9.e 10.b 11.e 12.b 13.b 14.c 15.d 16.c 17.c 18.a 19.d

LOCAL ANESTHETICS

Reference 1

20. **Vasoconstrictors reduce the systemic absorption of all of the following local anesthetics EXCEPT** : 397
a) Procaine
b) Prilocaine
c) Lidocaine
d) Mepivacaine

21. **Ester type of local anesthetics are hydrolysed by** : 397
a) Acetyl cholinesterase
b) Liver microsomal enzymes
c) Butyryl cholinesterase
d) All of these enzymes

22. **All of the following are long-acting local anesthetics EXCEPT** : 399
a) Chlorprocaine
b) Tetracaine
c) Bupivacaine
d) Etidocaine

23. **The onset of local anesthesia is sometimes accelerated by the use of** : 399
a) Vasoconstrictors
b) Vasodilators
c) Solutions saturated with carbon dioxide
d) Hyaluronidase

24. **All of the following local anesthetics depress the strength of cardiac contractions EXCEPT** : 401
a) Procaine
b) Mepivacaine
c) Etidocaine
d) Cocaine

25. The administration of large doses of which of the following local anesthetic can produce methemoglobinemia : 402

a) Bupivacaine
b) Mepivacaine
c) Prilocaine
d) Etidocaine

26. Which of the following local anesthetic is more likely to produce allergic reactions : 402

a) Prilocaine
b) Procaine
c) Mepivacaine
d) Lidocaine

Reference 2

27. Which of the following local anesthetic can cause ventricular tachycardia and fibrillation following systemic absorption : 337

a) Lidocaine
b) Procaine
c) Bupivacaine
d) Ropivacaine

28. The local anesthetic which has a very short half-life of about 25 sec. is : 339

a) Dibucaine
b) Lidocaine
c) Ropivacaine
d) Etidocaine
e) Chlorprocaine

29. Local anesthetic of choice for anesthesia of the cornea and conjunctiva is : 340

a) Dibucaine
b) Benzocaine
c) Tetracaine
d) Dyclonine

30. Sodium channels which are resistant to the blocking effect of tetrodotoxin are located in : 341

a) Vasomotor nerves
b) Smooth muscles
c) Cardiac myocytes
d) Respiratory smooth muscles

ANSWERS

20.b 21.c 22.a 23.c 24.d 25.c 26.b 27.c 28.e 29.c 30.c

SEDATIVES AND HYPNOTICS

Reference 1

31. **All of the following are sometimes referred to as "Sedative-autonomic" drugs EXCEPT :** 335

a) Hydroxyzine
b) Glutethimide
c) Imipramine
d) Chlorpheniramine

32. **Which of the following benzodiazepine is rapidly absorbed from the G.I.T. :** 335

a) Diazepam
b) Oxazepam
c) Temazepam
d) Triazolam

33. **The sedative-hypnotic which has the slowest onset of action is :** 335

a) Diazepam
b) Chlordiazepoxide
c) Meprobamate
d) Lorazepam

34. **The sedative-hypnotic which increases the anticoagulant effect of warfarin by displacing it from binding sites on plasma proteins is :** 336

a) Flurazepam
b) Phenobarbitone
c) Glutethimide
d) Chloral hydrate

35. **All of the following benzodiazepines are metabolised to active metabolites in the body EXCEPT :** 336

a) Chlordiazepoxide
b) Lorazepam
c) Chlorazepate
d) Flurazepam

36. **All of the following drugs facilitate or mimic the action of GABA by binding to chloride channel GABA receptor complex EXCEPT :** 338

a) Phenobarbitone
b) Diazepam
c) Propofol
d) Invermectin
e) Bicuculline
f) Alphaxolone

37. **The enhancement in chloride ion conductance by the interaction of benzodiazepines with GABA receptor results in :** 339

a) Increase in the duration of GABA gated channel openings
b) Increase in the frequency and reduced duration of channel openings

c) Increase in the frequency of channel opening events
d) Increase in duration and reduced frequency of channel openings

38. **The agent which acts as inverse agonist at benzodiazepine receptor is :** 339
a) Flurazepam
b) Beta-carbolines
c) Flumazenil
d) Bicuculine

39. **All of the following benzodiazepines have selective actions that are clinically useful in the management of seizure states EXCEPT :** 341
a) Diazepam
b) Nitrazepam
c) Oxazepam
d) Clonazepam
e) Lorazepam

40. **The effect of sedative hypnotic on the pattern of normal sleep includes all of the following EXCEPT :** 340
a) Latency of sleep onset is decreased
b) Duration of slow wave sleep is decreased
c) Duration of stage 2 NREM sleep is increased
d) Duration of REM sleep is decreased
e) Nocturnal peaks in LH are abolished

41. **Pharmacological effects of Buspirone include all of the following EXCEPT :** 342
a) It relieves anxiety without marked sedation
b) It has no hypnotic, anticonvulsant or muscle relaxant actions
c) It potentiates the CNS depressant actions of ethanol
d) It acts as a partial agonist at $5HT_{1A}$ receptors

Reference 2

42. **All of the following effects of benzodiazepines result from actions on the CNS EXCEPT :** 364
a) Sedation and hypnosis
b) Decreased anxiety
c) Coronary vasodilatation
d) Muscle relaxation
e) Anterograde amnesia
f) Anticonvulsant effect

43. **Although effective as anticonvulsant, benzodiazepines have limited use in the treatment of seizure disorders because :** 365
a) They are erratically absorbed from the GIT
b) They have short duration of action needing repeated administration
c) Tolerance to their anticonvulsant action develops rapidly
d) All of the above

44. **Zolipidem, a nonbenzodiazepine sedative hypnotic, differs from the benzodiazepines in all of the following respects EXCEPT :** 371

a) It produces only weak anticonvulsant action
b) It has similar effects on sleep stages as benzodiazepines
c) It has relatively strong sedative actions
d) Development of tolerance and physical dependence is seen only rarely

45. **The risk of occurrence of seizures is especially high if Flumazenil is given to patients poisoned with :** 373

a) Benzodiazepines
b) Barbiturates
c) Ethanol
d) Tricyclic antidepressants

46. **As tolerance develops to the effects of barbiturates the therapeutic index :** 374

a) Increases
b) Decreases
c) Remains unchanged
d) None of these

47. **Phenobarbitone causes induction of :** 377

a) Microsomal enzymes
b) Mitochondrial enzymes
c) Cytoplasmic enzymes
d) All of these enzymes

48. **Which of the following drug should be avoided in patients with intermittent porphyria as it causes induction of ALA synthetase enzyme :** 381

a) Glutethimide
b) Meprobamate
c) Methyprilon
d) Chloral hydrate

49. **A very potent inhibitor of alcohol dehydrogenase is :** 350/R-I

a) Disulfiram
b) Metronidazole
c) Cefamendol
d) Fomepizole
e) Albendazole

50. **Ethyl alcohol is converted to acetaldehyde by :** 350/R-I

a) Alcohol dehydrogenase present in the liver
b) Alcohol dehydrogenase present in the stomach
c) Microsomal ethanol oxidising enzymes
d) All of the above enzymes
e) Enzymes a and b

51. **The main pathway of acetaldehyde oxidation is :** 351/R-I

a) Cytoplasmic aldehyde dehydrogenase
b) Microsomal aldehyde dehydrogenase

c) Mitochondrial aldehyde dehydrogenase

d) Plasma aldehyde dehydrogenase

52. **One of the valuable markers of excess alcohol consumption and predisposition to alcoholism is alteration in the activity of :** 351/R-1

a) Na^+/K^+ ATPase

b) Adenyl cyclase in the platelets

c) 5^1-nucleotidase

d) RBC acetyl cholinesterase

53. **Chronic alcohol abuse can cause all of the following types of anemias EXCEPT :** 353/R-1

a) Megaloblastic anemia

b) Iron deficiency anemia

c) Hemolytic anemia

d) Sideroblastic anemia

54. **All of the following drugs have been studied as potential "prophylactic" agents that would decrease the craving for Ethanol EXCEPT :** 357/R-1

a) Fluoxetin

b) Bromocriptin

c) Nalaxone

d) Naltrexone

e) Tiapride

55. **Disulfiram irreversibly inhibits which form of aldehyde dehydrogenase :** 391/R-2

a) Cytosolic

b) Mitochondrial

c) Both cytosolic and mitochondrial

d) None of these enzymes

56. **Hypotension produced during disulfiram-ethanol interaction is due to:**391/R-2

a) Reduced release of noradrenaline from nerve endings

b) Inhibition of dopamine beta hydroxylase

c) Blockade of Alpha adrenergic receptors

d) Reduced central sympathetic outflow

ANSWERS

31.b 32.d 33.c 34.d 35.b 36.e 37.c 38.b 39.c 40.e 41.c 42.c 43.c 44.b 45.d 46.b 47.d 48.c 49.d 50.d 51.c 52.b 53.c 54.c 55.c 56.b

ANTIEPILEPTIC DRUGS

Reference 1

57. **Which of the following drug exerts its action by blocking T-type of calcium channels :** 361

a) Phenytoin

b) Carbamezapine
c) Ethosuximide
d) Valproic acid
e) Phenobarbitone

58. **All of the following antiepileptic drugs have similar chemical structure EXCEPT :** 362
a) Phenobarbitone
b) Phenytoin
c) Ethosuximide
d) Trimethadione
e) Carbamezapine

59. **The antiepileptic drug which can displace other highly protein bound drugs and cause drug-drug interactions is :** 362
a) Ethosuximide
b) Valproic acid
c) Phenobarbitone
d) Carbamezapine

60. **All of the following drugs have a dose-dependent elimination pharmacokinetics EXCEPT :** 364, 65, 72
a) Phenytoin
b) Aspirin
c) Mephetoin
d) Alcohol
e) Valproic acid

61. **At low blood levels of phenytoin, the time required for reaching steady state concentration after every dosage change is :** 364
a) 5-7 days
b) 3-4 days
c) 1-2 days
d) 10-15 days

62. **Therapeutic blood levels of phenytoin for most patients is between (/ug/ml)** : 364
a) 20-30
b) 5-8
c) 10-20
d) 5-10

63. **Which of the following drug inhibits the metabolism of phenytoin resulting in increased steady state concentration when the two drugs are given together :** 365
a) Carbamezapine
b) Phenobarbitone
c) Phenylbutazone
d) Isoniazide

64. **Which of the following adverse effect occurs early and is not an indication for reduction of the dose, following phenytoin therapy :** 365

a) Diplopia
b) Ataxia
c) Gingival hyperplasia
d) Nystagmus
e) Lymphadenopathy

65. **The pharmacological effects of carbamezapine include all of the following EXCEPT** : 365-67
a) It is effective in bipolar depression
b) It blocks sodium channels and inhibits high-frequency repetitive firing
c) It also acts presynaptically to decrease synaptic transmission
d) It inhibits uptake of GABA in brain slices
e) It inhibits uptake and release of norepinephrine from brain synaptosomes

66. **The irreversible inhibitor of GABA aminotransferase is** : 369
a) Phenobarbitone
b) Valproic acid
c) Vigabatrin
d) Lamotrigine

67. **The broad spectrum antiepileptic drug is** : 372
a) Phenobarbitone
b) Valproic acid
c) Gabapentin
d) Primidone

68. **Therapeutic plasma levels of valproic acid are between (/ug/ml)** : 373
a) 10-20
b) 20-30
c) 100-200
d) 50-100

69. **Which of the following drug can cause fulminating hepatotoxicity** : 373
a) Phenytoin
b) Methosuximide
c) Valproic acid
d) Bromides

70. **The antiepileptic drug that can cause Myasthenic syndrome as a toxic effect is** : 374
a) Ethosuximide
b) Trimethadione
c) Primidone
d) Ethotoin

71. **The drug which may have a special role in epileptic women who experience seizure exacerbation at the time of menstrual period is** : 375
a) Bromides
b) Clonazepam
c) Lorazepam
d) Acetazolamide

72. **The drug of choice for the treatment of infantile spasms is :** 377

a) Clonazepam

b) Nitrazepam

c) Corticotrophin

d) Vigabatrin

Reference 2

73. **All of the following drugs can cause an increase in the plasma concentration of phenytoin, when given together, EXCEPT :** 470

a) Carbamezapine

b) Chloramphenicol

c) Dicumarol

d) Disulfiram

e) Cimetidine

f) Valproic acid

74. **The concurrent administration of which of the following two drugs can lead to absence status epilepticus :** 477

a) Sodium valproate and Ethosuximide

b) Sodium valproate and Clonazepam

c) Ethosuximide and Trimethadione

d) Ethosuximide and Clonazepam

e) Sodium valproate and Trimethadione

75. **All of the following antiepileptic drugs cause induction of hepatic microsomal enzymes EXCEPT :** 481

a) Carbamezapine

b) Phenytoin

c) Phenobarbitone

d) Primidone

e) Sodium valproate

76. **The drug which has been found effective in controlling seizures in Lennox-Gastaut syndrome is :** 481

a) Gabapentin

b) Lomatrigine

c) Felbamate

d) Vigabatrin

77. **For which of the following antiepileptic drug evidence for a teratogenic effect is greatest :** 484

a) Trimethadione

b) Valproic acid

c) Phenytoin

d) Carbamezapine

e) Phenobarbitone

ANSWERS

57.c 58.e 59.b 60.d 61.a 62.c 63.d 64.d 65.d 66.c 67.b 68.d 69.c 70.b 71.d 72.c 73.f 74.b 75.e 76.c 77.a

OPIOID ANALGESICS

Reference 1

78. **The most potent opioid agonist is :** 460
   a) Hydromorphone
   b) Etorphin
   c) Oxymorphone
   d) Fentanyl
   e) Sufantenil
79. **The opioid analgesic that can be given transdermally is :** 463
   a) Fentanyl
   b) Buprenorphine
   c) Oxymorphone
   d) Lavarphanol
80. **Opioid analgesics metabolised by tissue esterases are :** 464
   a) Morphine
   b) Oxymorphone
   c) Meperidine
   d) Heroin
   e) Levarphanol
   f) Drugs a and b
   g) Drugs c and d
81. **Tolerance is not developed to all of the following actions of opioids EXCEPT :** 467
   a) Miosis
   b) Antidiuresis
   c) Constipation
   d) Convulsions
82. **The drug recently approved for detoxification and for maintenance of the chronic relapsing heroin addicts is :** 473
   a) Oxymorphone
   b) Methadone
   c) Levarphanol
   d) L-Alpha-acetyl-methadol
83. **The opioid analgesic whose effects are resistant to reversal by naloxone is :** 474
   a) Nalbufine
   b) Dezocine
   c) Buprenorphine
   d) Levarphanol

Reference 2

84. **Beta endorphin is found in the amino acid sequence of :** 522
   a) Melanocyte stimulating hormone
   b) Beta lipoprotein
   c) Adrenocorticotrophic hormone
   d) Proencephalin B

85. **The endogenous ligand for delta receptors is :** 525
   a) Beta endorphin
   b) Dynorphin B
   c) Enkephalins
   d) Dynorphin A

86. **The drug which irreversibly blocks Mu receptors is :** 523
   a) Naloxone
   b) Naltrexone
   c) Nalorphine Beta Funaltrexamine
   d) Beta Funaltrexamine

87. **All of the following effects result from the interaction of opioid agonists with Mu receptors EXCEPT :** 527
   a) Analgesia
   b) Amnesia
   c) Respiratory depression
   d) Miosis
   e) Euphoria

88. **Analgesia produced by morphine-like opioids is characterised by all of the following EXCEPT :** 529
   a) Sensory modalities other than pain are not affected
   b) Continuous dull pain is relieved better than sharp intermittent pain
   c) Nonciceptive and neuropathic pain are equally responsive
   d) Reaction to pain is altered by opioid analgesics
   e) The effect is partly due to inhibition of the release of neurotransmitters

89. **The effect of Mu receptor agonist on the GIT includes all of the following EXCEPT :** 532
   a) There is an increased secretion of gastric acid
   b) Gastric motility is decreased with prolongation of gastric emptying time
   c) The amplitude of nonpropulsive movements in the small intestine is increased
   d) Tone of the anal sphincter is greatly enhanced

90. **Most of the analgesic action of Morphine in patients receiving chronic oral medication with morphine is due to the formation of :** 534
   a) Morphine-3-glucuronide
   b) Morphine-6-glucuronide
   c) Normorphine
   d) Morphine-3-sulfate
   e) Morphine-6-sulfate

91. **Meperidine differs from morphine in all of the following respects EXCEPT :** 542
   a) It causes less constipation
   b) Rise in biliary pressure is less than morphine
   c) Therapeutic doses given during labour do not delay birth process
   d) It is conjugated in the liver to form corresponding glucuronide
   e) Toxic doses sometimes cause excitation of the CNS

92. **All of the following drugs are competitive Mu antagonists and exert their analgesic action by acting as agonists for K receptors EXCEPT :** 546
   a) Nalorphine
   b) Nalbuphine
   c) Cyclazocine
   d) Pentazocine

93. **A relatively selective antagonist for Kapa receptors is :** 549
   a) Nalmefene
   b) Naloxonazine
   c) Nor-binaltorphimine
   d) Naltrindole

ANSWERS

78.b 79.a 80.g 81.b 82.d 83.c 84.b 85.d 86.d 87.b 88.c 89.a 90.b 91.d 92.d 93.c

NONSTEROIDAL ANTI-INFLAMMATORY AGENTS, DRUGS USED IN GOUT

Reference 1

94. The concomitant use of which of the following drug has been shown to reduce the incidence of NSAID-induced gastrointestinal damage : 541
   a) Omeprazole
   b) Misoprostol
   c) Ranitidine
   d) Antacids

95. All of the following drugs procedures can be used to reduce fever during viral infections in children EXCEPT : 542
   a) Paracetamol
   b) Cold sponging
   c) Ibuprofen
   d) Aspirin

96. Aspirin reduces the pharmacological effects of all of the following drugs EXCEPT : 542
   a) Spironolactone
   b) Probenecid
   c) Tolbutamide
   d) Sulfinpyrazone

97. **The NSAID which possesses analgesic-anti-inflammatory effects but lacks antipyretic activity is :** 542

a) Paracetamol
b) Diflunisol
c) Tolmetin
d) Phenacetin

98. **The active metabolite of which of the following drug is somewhat selective in inhibiting COX-II enzyme :** 543

a) Phenacetin
b) Sulindac
c) Nabumatone
d) Phenylbutazone

99. **The NSAID reported to reduce synthesis of both prostaglandins and leukotrienes is :** 543

a) Aspirin
b) Indomethacin
c) Diclofenac
d) Ibuprofen
e) Drugs b and c
f) Drugs a and d

100. **NSAID with a very long half-life is :** 544

a) Ibuprofen
b) Diclofenac
c) Oxaprozin
d) Ketoprofen
e) Naproxen

101. **Indomethacin is indicated for the management of all of the following EXCEPT :** 545

a) Acute gout
b) Patent ductus arteriosus
c) Osteoarthritis
d) As an analgesic
e) Ankylosing spondylitis

102. **Indomethacin is preferred over other NSAID for the treatment of patent ductus arteriosus because :** 546

a) It is less toxic to premature newborn
b) It is more selective in inhibiting COX-II enzyme
c) It can be given intravenously
d) It inhibits the synthesis of both prostaglandins and leukotrienes

103. **Disease-modifying antirheumatic drugs include all of the following EXCEPT :** 547

a) Azathioprine
b) Penicillamine
c) Hydroxychloroquine
d) Carprofen
e) Gold salts

104. **Antimalarials have been used successfully, for their anti-inflammatory action, in all of the following conditions EXCEPT :** 548

a) Rheumatoid arthritis
b) Psoriatic arthritis
c) Juvenile chronic arthritis
d) Systemic lupus erythematosus

105. **The blunting of taste perception following therapy with penicillamine is due to the chelation of :** 550

a) Copper
b) Calcium
c) Iron
d) Zinc
e) Magnesium

106. **The analgesic-antipyretic drug which lacks an effect on platelets and uric acid levels is :** 552

a) Ibuprofen
b) Diflunisol
c) Paracetamol
d) Sulindac

Reference 2

107. **The inhibition of the enzyme COX-II is thought to mediate all of the following effects of NSAID EXCEPT :** 612

a) Antipyretic action
b) Gastric ulcer production
c) Analgesic action
d) Anti-inflammatory effect

108. **Of the available anti-inflammatory agents which of the following drug is known to interefere with the synthesis and/or actions of Cytokines like IL-l or TNF :** 619

a) Aspirin
b) Penicillamine
c) Methotrexate
d) Corticosteroids
e) Phenylbutazone

109. **NSAID are able to reduce fever induced by all of the following EXCEPT :** 620

a) Tissue damage
b) Inflammation
c) Prostaglandins given to women as abortifacient
d) Malignancy

110. **The drug which preferentially inhibits COX-II enzyme is :** 621

a) Nabumetone
b) Sulindac

c) Etodolac

d) Oxaprozin

111. **Which of the following NSAID is capable of antagonizing certain effects of prostaglandins : 635**

a) Sulindac

b) Meclofenamic acid

c) Etodolac

d) Tolmetin

112. **Which of the following anti-inflammatory drug has been frequently used to enhance the performance of race-horses : 642**

a) Tolmetin

b) Nabumetone

c) Oxaprozin

d) Phenylbutazone

113. **The NSAID which is only a weak inhibitor of cyclooxygenase and a potent uricosuric agent is : 643**

a) Aspirin

b) Diclofenac

c) Apazone

d) Nabutnetone

114. **The drug which is particularly useful in patients who have allergic hypersensitivity reactions to Aspirin is : 644**

a) Sulindac

b) Mefenamic acid

c) Tolmetin

d) Nimesulide

115. **Which of the following drug selectively inhibits 5-lipooxygenase or cystenil leukotriene receptor : 644**

a) Zileuton

b) Docebenzone

c) Piripost

d) All of the above

e) Drugs a and c

116. **Colchicine is useful in all of the following conditions EXCEPT : 649**

a) Acute gout

b) Prevention of attacks of familial Mediterranean fever

c) As analgesic-antipyretic

d) Primary biliary cirrhosis

e) Psoriasis

ANSWERS

94.b 95.d 96.c 97.b 98.c 99.e 100.c 101.d 102.c 103.d 104.b 105.d 106.c 107.b 108.d 109.c 110.a 111.b 112.d 113.c 114.d 115.d 116.c

ANTIPSYCHOTIC DRUGS

Reference 1

117. **The major metabolite of which of the following antipsychotic drug is more potent than the parent compound and accounts for most of its antipsychotic effects :** 433

a) Chlorpromazine
b) Thioridazine
c) Haloperidol
d) Fluphenazine

118. **Which of the following antipsychotic drug is likely to produce a very high incidence of extrapyramidal toxicity :** 435

a) Chlorpromazine
b) Perfenazine
c) Flufenazine
d) Haloperidol
e) Clozapine

119. **The incidence of sedative effect is high with which of the following antipsychotic drug :** 435

a) Flufenazine
b) Chlorpromazine
c) Molindone
d) Thiothixene

120. **The characteristics of D-2 receptor include all of the following EXCEPT :** 435

a) It is coded on chromosomes
b) It is found both pre and post synaptically
c) It increases cyclic AMP formation
d) It blocks calcium channels
e) It opens potassium channels

121. **The ability of antipsychotic drugs to act as dopamine antagonists explains all of their following effects EXCEPT :** 435

a) Antipsychotic action
b) Ability to produce Parkinsonian symptoms
c) Hyperprolactinemia
d) Tardive dyskinasia
e) Changes in eating habits

122. **The antipsychotic drug which acts exclusively on D-2 receptors is :** 436

a) Chlorpromazine
b) Pimozide
c) Thioridazine
d) Clozapine

123. **Indications for the use of antipsychotic drugs include all of the following EXCEPT :** 437

a) Schizophrenia
b) Maniac episode of bipolar affective disorder

c) Tourette's syndrome
d) Opioid withdrawal

124. **All of the following antipsychotic drugs have a strong antiemetic effect EXCEPT :** 438
a) Chlorpromazine
b) Prochlorpromazine
c) Thioridazine
d) Benzquinamide

125. **The antipsychotic drug which is most likely to produce agranulocytosis is :** 440
a) Thioridazine
b) Haloperidol
c) Flufenazine
d) Clozapine
e) Raclopride

126. **The antipsychotic drug which causes retinal deposits and "Browning" of vision is :** 440
a) Thioridazine
b) Chlorpromazine
c) Remoxipride
d) Pimozide

127. **All of the following drugs can be considered as "mood stabilizing" agents EXCEPT :** 442
a) Lithium
b) Carbamazepine
c) Sodium valproate
d) Oxazepam
e) Clonazepam

128. **The probable mechanism of action of Lithium includes all of the following EXCEPT :** 442-43
a) It enhances some of the actions of serotonin
b) It decreases norepinephrine and dopamine turnover
c) It blocks the development of dopamine supersensitivity
d) It increases norepinephrine sensitive adenyl cyclase levels
e) It augments Acetylcholine synthesis by increasing uptake of choline
f) It inhibits recycling of inositol substrates causing depletion of second messenger source of PIP_2

129. **The desired lithium concentration for the control of Bipolar affective disorder is :** (meq/L) 443
a) 0.6-1.4
b) 0.1-0.3
c) 3.0-4.0
d) 2.0-3.0

130. **All of the following drugs can reduce renal clearance of Lithium EXCEPT :** 444

a) Thiazides
b) Aspirin
c) Ibuprofen
d) Naproxen
e) Indomethacin

131. **The most frequent side-effect of lithium therapy is :** 444
a) Edema
b) Nephrogenic diabetes insipidus
c) Mental confusion
d) Tremor
e) Aphasia

Reference 2

132. **Pharmacological effects of Clozapine include all of the following EXCEPT :** 408-10
a) It has a dose-related risk of inducing seizures in nonepileptic patients
b) It has low affinity for D-2 receptors
c) It increases the secretion of prolactin in human beings
d) It is an active alpha-1 receptor blocking agent

133. **The pharmacological effect of Chlorpromazine on the pupil is characterised by :** 412
a) Miosis and blurring of vision
b) Mydriasis and blurring of vision
c) Mydriasis followed by miosis
d) Miosis with spasm of accommodation
e) Miosis followed by mydriasis

134. **The neurological syndromes which occur soon after the administration of anti-psychotic drugs include all of the following EXCEPT :** 414
a) Acute dystonia
b) Rabbit syndrome
c) Akathesia
d) Parkinsonism
e) Neuroleptic malignant syndrome

ANSWERS

117.b 118.d 119.b120.c 121.d 122.b 123.d 124.c 125.d 126.a 127.d 128.d 129.a 130.b 131.d 132.c 133.a 134.b

ANTI-DEPRESSANTS

Reference 1

135. **The antidepressant drug which is a highly selective serotonin uptake inhibitor is :** 450

a) Phenelzine
b) Imipramine
c) Fluoxetine
d) Doxepin

136. **The short-acting, selective MAO-A inhibitor is :** 451
a) Moclobemide
b) Isoniazide
c) Phenelzine
d) Tranylcypromine

137. **The antidepressant with shortest half-life is :** 451
a) Amoxapine
b) Imipramine
c) Doxepine
d) Trazodone
e) Paroxetin

138. **The antidepressant with a combined antidepressant and antipsychotic action is :** 453
a) Amitriptyline
b) Trazodone
c) Amoxapine
d) Proxetine

139. **The antidepressant drug which causes least degree of sedation is :** 454
a) Amitriptyline
b) Doxepine
c) Trazodone
d) Protryptaline

140. **The MAO inhibitor which is less likely to cause hypertensive crisis following ingestion of tyramine-containing food is :** 453
a) Phenelzine
b) Moclobemide
c) Isocarboxizide
d) Tranylcypromine

141. **All of the following antidepressants possess antimuscarinic effects EXCEPT :** 454
a) Amitriptyline
b) Paroxetine
c) Amoxepine
d) Doxepine
e) Maprotyline

ANSWERS

135.c 136.a 137.d 138.c 139.c 140.b 141.b

6

CHAPTER 8

HORMONES

THYROID AND ANTITHYROID DRUGS

Reference 1

1. **The major site of conversion of Thyroxin to Tri-iodothyronin is :** 1367
   a) Kidney
   b) Liver
   c) Lungs
   d) GIT
   e) Plasma
2. **Most tissues utilise tri-iodothyronin that is derived from circulating hormone EXCEPT :** 1388
   a) Brain
   b) Kidney
   c) Lungs
   d) Brain and Pituitary
   e) Heart
3. **Type I Iodothyronin-5′-deiodinase, which converts Thyroxin to Tri-iodothyronin is present in :** 1388
   a) Pitutary
   b) Placenta
   c) Liver, Kidney and Thyroid
   d) Heart
   e) Brain
4. **Type II Iodothyronin-5′-deiodinase is present in :** 1388
   a) Heart
   b) Lungs
   c) Brain
   d) Skin
   e) Kidney

5. **Type III, Iodothyronin-5′-deiodinase,which forms reverse Tri-iodothyronin is present in :** 1388

a) Brain

b) GIT

c) Kidney

d) Placenta

e) Sites a and d

f) Sites b and c

6. **Drugs which increase the binding of thyroxin to thyroxin-binding globulin include all of the following EXCEPT :** 1389

a) Estrogens

b) Methadone

c) Tamoxifen

d) Clofibrate

e) Carbamezapine

7. **Drugs which decrease the binding of thyroxin to thyroxin-binding globulin include all of the following EXCEPT :** 1389

a) Glucocorticoids

b) Androgens

c) 5-flurouracil

d) L-asparginase

e) Furosemide

8. **The activity of which of the following Iodothyronin-5′-deiodinase is affected by propylthiouracil :** 1388

a) Type I

b) Type II

c) Type III

d) All of the above

9. **The half-life of Tri-iodothyronin is :** 1389

a) 7 days

b) 1 day

c) 3 days

d) 4 days

10. **The recommended iodine content of iodised salt for prevention of Goiter in India is :** 1391

a) 15 ppm.

b) 30 ppm

c) 50 ppm

d) 100 ppm

11. **Which of the following tissue is unresponsive to the calorigenic response of thyroid hormone :** 1393

a) Heart

b) Skeletal muscle

c) Gonads
d) Liver
e) Kidney

12. **Indications for the use of thyroid hormone include all of the following EXCEPT :** 1395
a) Hypothyroidism
b) Sick euthyroid syndrome
c) Cretinism
d) For TSH suppression in nontoxic goiter

13. **The drug which acts as a potent inhibitor of iodotyrosine deiodination is :** 1397
a) Amiodarone
b) Phenytoin
c) Iodides
d) Sulfonamides

14. **The drug which is preferred for the treatment of hyperthyroidism during pregnancy is :** 1401
a) Carbimazole
b) Methimazole
c) Iodides
d) Propyl thiouracil

15. **The drug used for the treatment of amiodarone-induced thyrotoxicosis is :** 1401
a) Iodides
b) Perchlorate
c) Propylthiouracil
d) Radio active iodine
e) Methimazole

16. **The drug which decreases secretion of thyroxin and tri-iodothyronin is :** 1402
a) Perchlorate
b) Fluoborate
c) Lithium
d) Thiocyananate
e) Iodide

17. **The time required for 99% disappearance of radiation effect after I^{131} is :** 1404
a) 7 days
b) 14 days
c) 56 days
d) 32 days
e) 24 days

18. **The advantages of radioactive iodine therapy with I^{131} include all of the following EXCEPT :** 1405
a) No tissues other than thyroid is affected
b) Cost of therapy is low
c) No hospitilisation is required

d) Rapid control of hyperthyroidism is achieved

e) No death as a result of exposure to isotope is reported

19. **Indications for the use of radioactive iodine include all of the following EXCEPT :** 1405

a) Metastatic thyroid carcinoma

b) Patients above the age of 40 yrs.

c) Patients with heart disease

d) Toxic nodular goiter

e) Hyperthyroidism during pregnancy

f) Recurrence of hyperthyroidism after subtotal thyroidectomy

ANSWERS

1.b 2.d 3.c 4.c 5.e 6.e 7.c 8.b 9.b 10.a 11.c 12.b 13.a 14.d 15.b 16.c 17.c 18.d 19.e

ESTROGENS AND PROGESTINS

Reference 2

20. **Non-steroidal estrogens include all of the following EXCEPT :** 1412

a) Dinesterol

b) Diethylstilbesterol

c) Benzasterol

d) Mestranol

e) Methesterol

21. **Metabolic effects of estrogens include all of the following EXCEPT :** 1418

a) They block reabsorption and cause small increase in bone formation

b) They increase the level of hydroxylase which converts vitamin D to D_3

c) They increase plasma HDL levels and decrease LDL levels

d) They increase plasma levels of thyroxin-binding globulin

e) They decrease saturation of bile with cholesterol

22. **When given by transdermal route,estrogen have minimum effect on :** 1419

a) Bone tissue

b) Hydroxylase enzyme

c) Lipoprotein profile

d) Steroid-binding globulin

23. **The dose of estrogens used for postmenopausal replacement therapy is :** 1421

a) More than that used in oral contraceptives

b) Less than that used in oral contraceptives

c) Same as that used in oral contraceptives

d) Dose of natural estrogen is more, while that of synthetic estrogen is less

24. **The progestin most commonly used in hormone replacement regimens is :** 1423

a) Norethindrone

b) Norgestril

c) Medroxyprogesterone
d) Norethynodrel

25. **When used for the therapy of Turner's syndrome, estrogens replicate all the events of puberty EXCEPT :** 1423
a) Genital growth
b) Breast development
c) Axillary and pubic hair growth
d) Growth spurt and changes in the ovary
e) Feminine contour

26. **The time required for reaching steady state plasma levels after Tamoxifen is :** 1425
a) 1-2 weeks
b) 3-4 weeks
c) 4-11 days
d) 7-14 hours

27. **The progestin reported to have least androgenic activity is :** 1427
a) Desogestril
b) Norgestril
c) Norethindrone
d) Norethynodrel

28. **All of the following progestins bind to sex steroid binding globulin EXCEPT :** 1429
a) Norethindrone
b) Norgestrel
c) Desogestrel
d) Progesterone

29. **The drug which acts as a potent antagonist of both progesterone and glucocorticoid for binding to their respective receptors is :** 1430
a) Tamoxifen
b) Danazol
c) Clomiphene
d) Mifepristone

30. **Potential uses of Mifepristone include all of the following EXCEPT :** 1431
a) Postcoital contraceptive
b) Threatened abortion
c) Endometriosis
d) Meningiomas
e) Leiomyomas

31. **The estrogenic preparation most commonly employed in combination oral contraceptives is :** 1432-33
a) Mestranol
b) Estradiol
c) Ethinyl estradiol
d) Quinesterol

32. **Biphasic and Triphasic preparations of combination oral contraceptives were developed to :** 1432

a) Reduce the dose of estrogen given
b) Reduce the dose of progestins given
c) Both of these
d) None of these

33. **The mechanism of action of combination oral contraceptives include all of the following EXCEPT :** 1434

a) They inhibit ovulation by suppressing the levels of LH and FSH
b) Progesterone component diminishes the frequency of GnRH pulses
c) They increase pituitary responsiveness to GnRH
d) They interfere with the tubal transport of fertilised ovum and proper development of endometrium for implantation
e) They change the consistency and properties of cervical mucus which are important for sperm survival and penetration

34. **The most important mechanism of action of progestin-only contraceptive is :** 1434

a) Inhibition of ovulation
b) Slowing the frequency of GnRH pulses
c) Blunting of the LH surge
d) Thickening of cervical mucus and endometrial alteration which impairs sperm penetration and implantation

35. **Which of the following agent is likely to decrease the effectiveness of low-dose pills by reducing their enterohepatic recycling :** 1436

a) Rifampin
b) Phenytoin
c) Phenobarbitone
d) Tetracycline
e) Erythromycin
f) Cephalosporins

36. **As regards the relationship between oral contraceptives and cancer which of the following statement is most appropriate :** 1435

a) They increase the incidence of ovarian cancer
b) There is a small decrease in the incidence of hepatic adenoma
c) They decrease the incidence of endometrial cancer
d) There have been reports of decreased rates of cervical cancer
e) Their use around the time of menopause may decrease the risk of breast cancer

ANSWERS

20.d 21.e 22.c 23.b 24.c 25.d 26.b 27.a 28.d 29.d 30.b 31.c 32.b 33.c 34.d 35.d 36.c

ANDROGENS

Reference 2

37. **The metabolite of testosterone which serves as the intracellular mediator of most action of the hormone is :** 1442

a) Androstenedione
b) Dihydrotestosterone
c) Androsterone
d) Dehydroepiandrosterone

38. **Testosterone undecanoate is effective orally because :** 1442

a) It is slowly metabolised in the liver
b) It is absorbed via the lymphatic ducts rather than portal system
c) It is absorbed mainly from the upper part of the rectum
d) It is secreted in the saliva from where it is reabsorbed in systemic circulation

39. **The anabolic effects of androgens are more pronounced in all of the following EXCEPT :** 1445

a) Hypogonadal men
b) Women
c) Boys before puberty
d) Normal men

40. **5-Alpha reductase I, which converts testosterone to dihydrotestosterone, is located in :** 1446

a) Kidney
b) Uro-genital tract
c) Liver and nongenital skin
d) GIT

41. **In one form of pseudohermaphroditism, the target tissues are deficient in :** 1446

a) 5-alpha reductase II
b) 5-alpha reductase I
c) GnRH
d) None of the above enzymes

42. **The ultra-long-acting ester of testosterone is :** 1446

a) Testosterone propionate
b) Testosterone cypionate
c) Testosterone enathate
d) Testosterone buciclate

43. **Because it is a poor substrate for the aromatase enzyme, feminization is not a side-effect of which of the following androgen :** 1450

a) Testosterone
b) Danazol
c) Fluoxymesterone
d) Oxandrolone

44. **The feminizing side-effects of androgens are particularly severe in men with :** 1450

a) Heart disease
b) Liver disease
c) Kidney disease
d) Prostatic cancer

45. **Disturbances of hepatic function have not been reported with which of the following preparations of androgens :** 1450
a) Danazol
b) Fluoxymesterone
c) Methyltestosterone
d) Testosterone esters

46. **Androgenic and anabolic effects of androgens result from :** 1451
a) Different actions of same hormone
b) Same action of the hormone in different tissues
c) Different actions of different hormones
d) Same action of different hormones

47. **The androgen effective in hereditary angioneurotic edema is :** 1452
a) Testosterone
b) Testosterone propionate
c) Danazol
d) Testosterone cypionate

48. **Inhibitors of androgen synthesis include all of the following EXCEPT :** 1453
a) Spironolactone
b) Ketoconazole
c) Finestiride
d) Lioprolide
e) Liorazole

49. **A nonsteroidal antiandrogen that is devoid of other hormonal activity is :** 1453
a) Cyproterone
b) Flutamide
c) Finasteride
d) Spironolactone

ANSWERS

37.b 38.b 39.d 40.c 41.a 42.d 43.c 44.b 45.d 46.b 47.c 48.c 49.b

CORTICOSTEROIDS

Reference 1

50. **All the effects of corticosteroids can be explained on the basis of gene expression, after their interaction with glucocorticoid response element EXCEPT :** 594
a) Effect on carbohydrate metabolism
b) Effect on protein metabolism

c) Feedback inhibition of ACTH
d) Effect on water and electrolyte metabolism

51. **Metabolic effects of glucocorticoids include all of the following EXCEPT :** 594
a) Increased neoglucogenesis
b) Decreased glycogen deposition
c) Inhibition of uptake of glucose by fat cells
d) Increased breakdown of protein
e) Increased lipolysis and redistribution of fat

52. **Glucocorticoids decrease the number of all of the following blood elements EXCEPT :** 594
a) Eosinophils
b) Lymphocytes
c) Basophils
d) Neutrophils
e) Monocytes

53. **Corticosteroid induced myopathy is most likely to occur after the use of :** 600
a) Hydrocortisone
b) Triamcinolone
c) Dexamethasone
d) Prednisolone

Reference 2

54. **The rate-limiting step in the synthesis of steroid hormones is :** 1461
a) Conversion of Pregnenolone to Progesterone
b) Conversion of Progesterone to 17-Alpha Hydroxyprogesterone
c) Conversion of 11-deoxycortisol to cortisol
d) Conversion of Cholesterol to Pregnenolone

55. **The effect of corticosteroids on electrolyte metabolism include all of the following EXCEPT :** 1469
a) Increased reabsorption of sodium from tubular fluid
b) Decreased excretion of calcium
c) Increased excretion of potassium
d) Decreased absorption of calcium from the gut

56. **Corticosteroids increase vascular reactivity to other vasoactive substances by :** 1469
a) Retention of salt and water
b) Increased release of noradrenaline from nerve endings
c) Increased expression of adrenergic receptors in the vascular wall
d) All of the above

57. **In primary hyperaldosteronism muscle weakness results mainly from :** 1470
a) Hypokalemia
b) Muscle wasting

c) Inadequacy of circulatory system

d) Decreased release of acetylcholine at NMJ

58. **Chemical modification of cortisol molecule have resulted in the production of corticosteroid which differ from the parent compound in all of the following respects EXCEPT :** 1472-73

a) Separation of mineralocorticoid and glucocorticoid activity

b) Greater potency of compounds

c) Longer duration of action

d) Separation of anti-inflammatory and metabolic effects

59. **All of the following are 9-alpha-fluro derivatives of cortisol with potent glucocorticoid activity EXCEPT :** 1475

a) Fludrocortisone

b) Prednisone

c) Triamcinolone

d) Betamethasone

60. **The age group which is at particular risk of developing cataract after prolonged therapy with glucocorticoid is :** 1476

a) Males between 20-30 yrs

b) Females between 30-40 yrs

c) Children

d) Men and women above 50 yrs

61. **Osteoporosis following therapy with corticosteroids is due to all of the following EXCEPT :** 1476

a) Inhibition of the activity of osteoblasts decreasing bone formation

b) Inhibition of calcium absorption from the GIT

c) Increased calcium excretion by the kidney

d) Decreased parathyroid hormone secretion

62. **Glucocorticoids are used in all of the following conditions EXCEPT :** 1479

a) Rheumatoid arthritis

b) Nephrotic syndrome

c) Anaphylaxis

d) H.influenze meningitis in infants and children

e) Herpes simplex keratitis

63. **The drug which inhibits the conversion of cholesterol into pregnenolone is :** 1482

a) Ketoconazole

b) Aminoglutethimide

c) Metyrapone

d) Mitotane

64. **A competitive reversible inhibitor of the enzyme which converts pregnenolone to progesterone is :** 1482

a) Mitotane

b) Metyrapone

c) Aminoglutathemide

d) Ketoconazole
e) Trilostane

65. **Metyrapone inhibits the enzyme :** 1476
a) P-450 cholesterol side-chain cleavage enzyme
b) The enzyme that carries out betahydroxylation of steroids
c) Aromatase enzyme which converts androgens to estrogens
d) 3-beta-hydroxysteroid dehydrogenase

ANSWERS

50.c 51.b 52.d 53.b 54.d 55.b 56.c 57.a 58.d 59.b 60.c 61.d 62.e 63.b 64.e 65.b

ANTIDIABETIC DRUGS

Reference 1

66. **Type I Diabetes is characterised by all of the following EXCEPT :** 637
a) It occurs commonly in juveniles
b) Circulating Insulin is absent
c) Plasma Glucagon is reduced
d) Beta cells fail to respond to all insulogenic stimuli

67. **Beta cells of the pancreas secrete all of the following EXCEPT :** 638
a) Insulin
b) Proinsulin
c) C-peptide
d) Islet amyloid polypetide
e) Pancreatic polypeptide

68. **Insulin Unit is presently defined on the basis of weight and current Insulin standards used for assay purposes contain :** (Units/mg) 638
a) 22 units
b) 28 units
c) 24 units
d) 30 units

69. **Quantitatively the most important glucose transporter (GLUT) in terms of lowering blood sugar level is :** 640
a) GLUT 2
b) GLUT 5
c) GLUT 4
d) GLUT 1
e) GLUT 3

70. **Production of which of the preparation of Insulin has recently been discontinued, as no clinical indication for its use exists :** 642
a) Lente Insulin
b) Ultralente Insulin

c) Isophane Insulin

d) Semilente Insulin

71. **Ultralente Insulin is prepared only from :** 642

a) Pork Insulin

b) Beef Insulin

c) Avian Insulin

d) South American guinea-pig Insulin

72. **Human Insulin has all of the following characteristics EXCEPT :** 644

a) It is as effective as animal insulin

b) It is less immunogenic

c) There is a higher risk of hypoglycemia

d) It is absorbed more rapidly and has a slightly longer duration of action

73. **Insulin secretion is inhibited by all of the following drugs EXCEPT :** 647

a) Somatostatin

b) Clonidine

c) Vinblastin

d) Colchicine

e) Isoprenaline

74. **The mechanism of action of Sulfonylureas involve all of the following EXCEPT :** 647

a) Increased release of Insulin due to decreased efflux of potassium

b) Reduction of serum glucagon levels

c) Increased synthesis of Insulin

d) Increased binding of Insulin to insulin receptors

75. **The safest sulfonylurea compound for use in elderly diabetics is :** 649

a) Chlorpropamide

b) Acetohexamide

c) Glyburide

d) Tolbutamide

76. **The oral hypoglycemic agent which can be termed as "euglycemic" agent rather than hypoglycemic agent is :** 651

a) Glipizide

b) Glyburide

c) Metformin

d) Tolazamide

77. **The mechanism of action of Biguanide derivatives include all of the following EXCEPT :** 651

a) Direct stimulation of glycolysis in peripheral tissues

b) Increased hepatic neoglucogenesis

c) Slowing of glucose absorption from GIT

d) Reduction of plasma glucagon levels

e) Increased binding of Insulin to receptors

78. **Pharmacological effects of Glucagon include all of the following EXCEPT :** 652

a) Glycogenolysis in the liver
b) Gluconeogenesis and ketogenesis
c) Glycogenolysis in the skeletal muscle
d) Release of insulin from the beta cells
e) Positive inotropic and chronotropic action on the heart

Reference : 2

79. **The first hormone for which a radioimmunoassay was developed was :** 1488
a) Thyroxin
b) Insulin
c) Growth hormone
d) Parathormone

80. **The endopeptidases responsible for the conversion of Proinsulin to Insulin are :** 1490
a) PC1 and Furin
b) PC2 and Furin
c) PC2 and PC3
d) PC3 and Furin
e) PC1 and PC3

81. **Insulin promotes glucose transport across the cell at least in part by :** 1492
a) Increasing phosphorylation of glucose
b) Promoting translocation of GLUT-4 to the plasma membrane
c) Promoting translocation of GLUT-7 to plasma membrane
d) Promoting translocation of GLUT-4 and GLUT-l to plasma membrane
e) Promoting translocation of GLUT-7 and GLUT-l to plasma membrane

82. **The hexokinase which promotes facilitated diffusion of glucose in the liver and pancreatic beta cells is :** 1492
a) Hexokinase IV
b) Hexokinase I
c) Hexokinase II
d) Hexokinase III

83. **Diabetes mellitus, which results from the mutation of Glucokinase gene, is known as :** 1494
a) Gestational diabetes
b) Tropical diabetes
c) Prader-Willi syndrome
d) Maturity onset diabetes of youth (MODY)
e) Insulin gene mutation diabetes

84. **NIDDM is characterised by all of the following EXCEPT :** 1495
a) Reduction of beta cell mass
b) "True" insulin values are no greater or distinctly less than values in control
c) Plasma proinsulin is increased
d) Responses to secretogogues (arginine) is reduced
e) Defect in first phase insulin secretion in response to an I.V. glucose dose

85. **Insulin concentration of 20/μg/ml produces all of the following responses EXCEPT :** 1496

a) Decreased gluconeogenesis
b) Stimulation of glucose uptake in the muscle
c) Decreased glycogenolysis
d) Stimulation of glucose uptake in the liver
e) Inhibition of hormone-sensitive lipase in adipose tissue

86. **After S.C. injection absorption of insulin is usually most rapid from :** 1502

a) Buttock
b) Arm
c) Thigh
d) Abdominal wall
e) Dorsal arm

87. **Neuroglycopenic symptoms of hypoglycemia include all of the following EXCEPT :** 1503

a) Difficulty in concentration
b) Confusion
c) Drowsiness
d) Paresthesias
e) Blurred vision

88. **Which of the following sulfonylureas is least bound to plasma proteins :** 1508

a) Chlorpropamide
b) Glyburide
c) Tolazamide
d) Tolbutamide
e) Acetohexamide

89. **Match the Drug given in Column A with the Mechanism of hypoglycemia in Column B :** 1505

Column A	Column B
1. Ethanol	a) Destruction of beta cells & insulin release
2. Propranolol	b) Inhibition of Gluconeogenesis
3. Salicylates	c) Increased sensitivity of beta cells to glucose
4. pentamidine	d) Inhibition of the effect of catecholamines on gluconeogenesis and glycogenolysis

90. **The insulin analogue which is being developed, as it retains the monomeric or dimeric configuration of native insulin is :** 1505

a) Lys(B29), Pro(B28) human insulin
b) Human proinsulin
c) Porcine proinsulin
d) Lys(B28), Pro(B29) human insulin

91. **The most promising new route of insulin delivery as an alternative to S.C. injection is :** 1506

a) Oral route
b) Intraperitoneal infusion
c) Subcutaneous pellets
d) Rectal pessary
e) Nasal spray

92. **The predominant form of somatostatin found in the brain is :** 1512
a) Somatostatin-28
b) Somatostatin-14
c) Somatostatin-28 (S-28,1-12)
d) All of the above

93. **Somatostatin inhibits the release of :** 1512
a) TSH
b) Growth hormone
c) Gastrin
d) VIP
e) Insulin and glucagon
f) All of the above
g) Hormones a, c, and e

94. **Adverse effect of Diazoxide which specially occurs in children is :** 1513
a) Retention of sodium
b) Hypertrichosis
c) Hyperuricemia
d) Leucopenia
e) Thrombocytopenia

95. **A long-acting analogue of Somatostatin-Octreotide, is used for the treatment of all of the following EXCEPT :** 1513
a) Carcinoid tumors
b) Glucagonomas
c) Acromegaly
d) Diarrhea in autonomic neuropathy
e) Gall stones
f) Bleeding esophageal verices
g) Postprandial orthostatic hypotension

96. **The mechanism of hyperglycemic effect of Diazoxide involves all of the following EXCEPT :** 1513
a) Inhibition of Insulin synthesis
b) Opening of potassium channels
c) Stimulation of hepatic gluconeogenesis
d) Inhibition of peripheral glucose utilization

ANSWERS

66.c 67.e 68.b 69.c 70.d 71.b 72.d 73.e 74.c 75.d 76.c 77.b 78.c 79.b 80.c 81.d 82.a 83.d 84.d 85.b 86.d 87.d 88.a 89.1=b, 2=d, 3=c, 4=a 90.d 91.e 92.b 93.f 94.b 95.e 96.a

DRUGS AFFECTING CALCIFICATION AND BONE TURNOVER

Reference 2

97. **All of the following agents act by preventing bone reabsorption rather than by promoting new bone formation EXCEPT :** 1519

a) Estrogens
b) Fluoride
c) Calcium
d) Calcitonin
e) Biophosphonates

98. **The drug which is absorbed by both active transport and facilitated diffusion is :** 1520

a) Iron
b) Glucose
c) L-DOPA
d) Calcium
e) Vitamin B-12

99. **All of the following agents are useful in the treatment of Hypercalcemia EXCEPT :** 1524

a) Corticosteroids
b) Calcitonin
c) Mithramycin
d) Etidronate
e) Edetate disodium
f) Gallium nitrate

100. **Physiological anemia of the childhood is probably due to :** 1524

a) Increased destruction of R.B.C.
b) Decreased number of R.B.C.
c) Hyperphosphatemia
d) Hypercalcemia

101. **Parathyroid hormone secretion is increased by all of the following EXCEPT :** 1527

a) Isoprenaline
b) Dopamine
c) Hypocalcemia
d) Hypomagnesemia

102. **The hormone which has no currently valid therapeutic use is :** 1529

a) Parathyroid hormone
b) Calcitonin
c) Thyroxin
d) Calcitriol

103. **Though termed as vitamin, which of the following functions as a hormone :** 1529

a) Vitamin A
b) Vitamin C

c) Folic acid
d) Vitamin D
e) Vitamin K

104. **The active constituent in the commercial Vitamin D preparations and in irradiated bread and milk is :** 1529
a) Ergocalciferol
b) Cholecalciferol
c) Calcifediol
d) Calcitriol

105. **The enzyme which converts calcifediol to calcitriol is present in all of the following EXCEPT :** 1530
a) Kidney
b) Macrophages
c) Placenta
d) Liver
e) Decidua

106. **Pharmacological effects of Parathyroid hormone include all of the following EXCEPT :** 1527
a) Increased overall bone resorption
b) Increased calcium reabsorption from kidney even at normal plasma calcium concentration
c) Inhibition of tubular reabsorption of phosphates
d) Stimulation of conversion of vitamin D to calcitriol
e) Reduction of concentration of calcium in milk and saliva

107. **The activity of 1-Alpha-hydroxylase which converts 25-OHD to calcitriol is increased by all of the following EXCEPT :** 1531
a) Low calcium and phosphate
b) Prolactin
c) Estrogens
d) Parathyroid hormone
e) Vitamin C

108. **Pharmacological effects of Calcitriol include all of the following EXCEPT :** 1532
a) Increased absorption of calcium from the small intestine
b) Mobilization of calcium from bones by a direct effect on mature osteoblast
c) Reduced excretion of calcium by the kidney
d) Inhibition of epidermal proliferation and promotion of epidermal differentiation

109. **Hypervitaminosis D is particularly dangerous in patients who are receiving :** 1533
a) Beta agonists
b) Beta blockers
c) Digitalis
d) Verapamil

110. **The agent of choice for maintaining normal plasma concentration of calcium in patients with hypoparathyroidism is :** 1534

a) Parathyroid hormone
b) Dihydrotachysterol
c) Ergocalciferol
d) Calcifediol
e) Calcitriol

111. **The compound which is being evaluated as a potential treatment for Psoriasis is :** 1534

a) Calcitriol
b) Ergocalciferol
c) Cholecalciferol
d) Calcipotriol
e) 22-oxacalcitriol

112. **The drug used for treating malignancy associated with hypercalcemia is :** 1524

a) Corticosteroids
b) Gallium nitrate
c) Pamidronate
d) Sodium phosphate
e) Calcitonin

ANSWERS

97.b 98.d 99.e l00.c l01.d 102.a 103.d 104.a 105.d 106.b 107.e 108.b 109.c 110.b 111.d 112.b

CHAPTER 9

ANTIMICROBIAL AGENTS

BETA LACTAM ANTIBIOTICS

Reference 1

1. **The mechanism of action of all the following antibiotics involves inhibition of cell wall synthesis EXCEPT :** 671

a) Penicillin
b) Bacitracin
c) Amikacin
d) Cycloserine
e) Vancomycin

2. **The mode of action of all the following antibiotics involves attachment to a specific receptor protein on 30 S subunit of the microbial ribosome EXCEPT :** 674-75

a) Gentamycin
b) Lincomycin
c) Netlmicin
d) Tetracyclines

3. **All of the following antibiotics produce their effect by attachment to 50 S subunit of ribosome EXCEPT :** 676-77

a) Ciprofloxacin
b) Chloramphenicol
c) Erythromycin
d) Clindamycin

4. **Inhibition of Nucleic acid synthesis is the mechanism of action of all of the following antimicrobial agents EXCEPT :** 677

a) Rifampin
b) Pyrimethamine
c) Trimethoprim
d) Cefotaxime
e) Ciprofloxacin

5. The preparation of choice for the prophylaxis and treatment of beta-hemolytic streptococcal pharyngitis is : 684

a) Crystalline penicillin
b) PAM
c) Procaine penicillin
d) Benzathine penicillin

6. Treatment of choice for H.Influenze meningitis is with : 684

a) Ampicillin
b) Ceftriaxone
c) Amoxycillin
d) Carbenicillin

7. The beta-lactam antibiotic which can cause interstitial nephritis is : 685

a) Dicloxacillin
b) Nafcillin
c) Methicillin
d) Ampicillin

8. All of the following cephalosporins are effective orally EXCEPT : 686-89

a) Cephalexin
b) Cefadroxil
c) Cefaclor
d) Cefuroxime
e) Cefotaxime

9. The First generation cephalosporin of choice for surgical prophylaxis is : 688

a) Cephalexin
b) Cefazolin
c) Cefadroxil
d) Cefradine

10. The only Second generation cephalosporin which crosses blood-brain barrier is : 688

a) Cefaclor
b) Cefamandole
c) Cefoxitin
d) Cefotetan
e) Cefuroxime

11. Third generation cephalosporins excreted mainly through bile are : 689

a) Cefoperazone
b) Cefotaxime
c) Ceftazidine
d) Ceftriaxone
e) Drugs a and d
f) Drugs b and c

12. Cephalosporins which can cause hypo-prothrombinemia and disulfiram like reactions include all of the following EXCEPT : 689

a) Cefamandole
b) Cefotetan
c) Cefoperazone
d) Cefotaxime
e) Cefmetazole

Reference 2

13. **One milligram of pure penicillin G sodium contains :** 1074
a) 1557 units
b) 1667 units
c) 1567 units
d) 1657 units

14. **All of the following penicillins are well absorbed orally EXCEPT :** 1078
a) Carbenicillin Indanyl
b) Ticarcillin
c) Amoxycillin
d) Dicloxacillin

15. **The drug of choice for the treatment of Methicillin resistant staphylococcal infection is :** 1083
a) Tetracycline
b) Erythromycin
c) Clindamycin
d) Vancomycin
e) Mezlocillin

16. **The Cephalosporin most resistant to staphylococcal beta-lactamase is :** 1093
a) Cephalothin
b) Cefalexin
c) Cefadroxil
d) Cefradine

17. **Cephalosporins which can be classified as Cephamycins are :** 1094
a) Cefaclor
b) Loracarbef
c) Cefoxitin
d) Cefuroxime
e) Cefotetan
f) Drugs a and d
g) Drugs c and e

18. **The Cephalosporin which is effective against B.fragilis is :** 1094
a) Cefotaxime
b) Cefoxitin
c) Ceftriaxone
d) Ceftazidime

19. **All of the following drugs are effective against B.fragilis EXCEPT :** 1094
   a) Clindamycin
   b) Metronidazole
   c) Chloramphenicol
   d) Cefotetan
   e) Cefotaxime

20. **A single dose of which of the following antibiotics is effective in the treatment of Gonorrhoea caused by Penicillinase producing microorganisms :** 1095
   a) Cefotaxime
   b) Ceftriaxone
   c) Cefoxitin
   d) Ceftazidine
   e) Moxalactam

ANSWERS

l.c 2.b 3.a 4.d 5.d 6.b 7.c 8.e 9.b 10.e 11.e 12.d 13.b 14.b 15.d 16.a 17.g 18.b 19.e 20.b

AMINOGLYCOSIDAL ANTIBIOTICS

Reference 2

21. **The semisynthetic aminoglycosidal antibiotic is :** 1104
   a) Kanamycin
   b) Gentamycin
   c) Amikacin
   d) Sisomycin

22. **All of the following are aminoglycosidic-aminocyclotols EXCEPT :** 1104
   a) Sisomycin
   b) Netlmicin
   c) Neomycin
   d) Spectinomycin
   e) Paromomycin

23. **The aminoglycosidal antibiotic effective against Cryptosporidiosis in AIDS patients is :** 1104
   a) Neomycin
   b) Paramomycin
   c) Amikacin
   d) Gentamycin
   e) Netilmicin

24. **The mechanism of development of resistance to aminoglycosides involves all of the following EXCEPT :** 1107
   a) Failure of the drug to penetrate through pores in the outer membrane

b) Absence of aminoglycosidal binding proteins in the organism
c) Production of drug inactivating enzymes
d) Alteration of the ribosomal structure

25. **Resistance to Gentamycin indicates resistance to all of the following EXCEPT :** 1107
a) Streptomycin
b) Tobramycin
c) Amikacin
d) Kanamycin
e) Netilmicin

26. **With regard to aminoglycosidal antibiotics, in patients with impaired renal function :** 1109
a) Loading dose of the drug should be reduced
b) Maintenance dose of the drug should be reduced
c) There is no need to change the dosage
d) Dosage should remain the same, but the interval between the dosages should be increased

27. **Half-life of the aminoglycosides is five to six times longer in the :** 1110
a) Cerebrospinal fluid
b) Aqueous humor
c) Prostatic fluid
d) Otic fluids

28. **The aminoglycosidal antibiotic which affects vestibular and auditory functions equally is :** 1111
a) Streptomycin
b) Gentamycin
c) Tobramycin
d) Amikacin
e) Kanamycin

29. **The least nephrotoxic aminoglycosidal antibiotic is :** 1112
a) Neomycin
b) Streptomycin
c) Gentamycin
d) Vancomycin
e) Amphotericin B

30. **The mechanism by which aminoglycosides produce neuromuscular blockade is :** 1113
a) Blockade of nicotinic receptors
b) Reduced release of acetylcholine from nerve endings
c) Reduced release of calcium from sarcoplasmic reticulum
d) Desensitization of nicotinic receptors
e) Blockade of impulse transfer from "T" tubules to sarcoplasmic reticulum

ANSWERS

21.c 22.d 23.b 24.b 25.a 26.b 27.d 28.c 29.b 30.b

CHLORAMPHENICOL, TETRACYCLINES, MACROLIDES

Reference 1

31. **The First completely synthetic antibiotic to be produced commercially was :** 693
    a) Penicillin V
    b) Doxycycline
    c) Erythromycin
    d) Chloramphenicol
32. **Aplastic anemia caused by Chloramphenicol has all of the following characteristics EXCEPT :** 694
    a) It is not related to dose
    b) It occurs when the drug is given orally
    c) It represents a specific genetically determined idiosyncrasy
    d) It is seen more frequently with prolonged use
    e) It tends to be irreversible and fatal
33. **Ability of chloramphenicol to prolong the half-life and raise blood concentration of Phenytoin and Tolbutamide is due to :** 694
    a) Displacement of these drugs from plasma proteins
    b) Reduced excretion of these drugs by the kidney
    c) Increased absorption and reduced excretion of these drugs
    d) Inhibition of liver microsomal enzymes
34. **The tetracycline which is completely absorbed from the GIT is :** 696
    a) Minocycline
    b) Demeclocycline
    c) Oxytetracycline
    d) Methacycline
35. **Absorption of tetracyclines from the GIT is impaired by all of the following EXCEPT :** 696
    a) Milk
    b) Antacids
    c) Presence of food
    d) Acidic pH
36. **The tetracycline which reaches a high concentration in tears and saliva is :** 696
    a) Doxycycline
    b) Minocycline
    c) Demeclocycline
    d) Methacycline
37. **A tetracycline which does not accumulate significantly in renal failure is :** 696
    a) Minocycline
    b) Demeclocyline

c) Chlotetracycline
d) Doxycycline

38. **The tetracycline which is effective in the treatment of syndrome of inappropriat-secretion of ADH is :** 696
a) Doxycycline
b) Minocycline
c) Demeclocycline
d) Methacycline

39. **Pseudomembranous colitis caused by tetracyclines is treated by giving :** 697
a) Oral Bacitracin
b) I.V. Vancomycin
c) Oral Spectinomycin
d) Oral Vancomycin

40. **Photodermatitis is most likely to occur with which of the following tetracycline :** 697
a) Minocycline
b) Demeclocycline
c) Oxytetracycline
d) Doxycycline

41. **The tetracycline which can cause vestibular paresis in children is :** 697
a) Tetracycline
b) Doxycycline
c) Demeclocycline
d) Minocycline

42. **The antibiotic used exclusively for treating gonorrhoea in patients who have contraindications to first line drugs is :** R2/1123
a) Doxycycline
b) Vancomycin
c) Spectinomycin
d) Erythromycin

Reference 2

43. **The most active congener of tetracyline is :** 1125
a) Doxycycline
b) Demeclocycline
c) Methacycline
d) Minocycline

44. **Food does not interfere with the absorption of which of the following tetracycline :** 1126
a) Demeclocycline
b) Chlotetracycline
c) Doxycycline
d) Methacycline

45. **Erythromycin is recommended for the treatment of all of the following EXCEPT :** 1139

a) Legionnaires' disease
b) Diphtheria
c) Resistant staphylococcal infection
d) Pertussis

46. **I.V. administration of Erythromycin can cause abdominal cramps, nausea, vomiting and diarrhea due to stimulation of :** 1140

a) Muscarinic receptors
b) H-l receptors
c) Motilin receptors
d) 5HT-l receptors

47. **A combination of Terfenadine and Erythromycin can rarely cause which of the following serious toxicities :** 1140

a) A-V block
b) Torsades de Pointes
c) Auditory impairment with loss of hearing
d) Hypertrophic pyloric stenosis

48. **The antibitoic which has some activity against Chloroquin-resistant strains of P.Vivax and P.Falciparum is :** 1141

a) Spectinomycin
b) Clarithromycin
c) Clindamycin
d) Vancomycin
e) Colistin

49. **The preferred treatment for brain abscess due to B.Fragilis is :** 1142

a) Cefoxitin
b) Chloramphenicol + penicillin
c) Clindamycin
d) Cefotaxime
e) Cefotaxime + Gentamycin

50. **Glycopeptide antimicrobial agents include all of the following EXCEPT :** 1143-44

a) Vancomycin
b) Polymyxin
c) Daptomycin
d) Teicoplanin

51. **The antibiotic produced by an actinomycete isolated from soil samples obtained from India is :** 1144

a) Colistin
b) Chloramphenicol
c) Vancomycin
d) Streptomycin

52. **"Red men Syndrome" is caused by the rapid I.V. infusion of which of the following antibiotic :** 1146

a) Vancomycin
b) Gentamycin
c) Polymyxin B
d) Cefotaxime

53. **Glycylcyclines are tetracycline derivatives which have been found to be effective against multidrug resistant :** 1148

a) Meningococci
b) Tubercle bacilli
c) Staphylococci
d) Gonococci

ANSWERS

31.d 32.b 33.d 34.a 35.d 36.b 37.d 38.c 39.d 40.b 41.d 42.c 43.a 44.c 45.c 46.c 47.b 48.c 49.b 50.b 51.c 52.a 53.c

SULFONAMIDES AND FLUOROQUINOLONES

Reference 1

54. **The microorganisms whose growth is stimulated by sulfonamides are :** 717

a) Staphylococci
b) Nocardia
c) Rickettsiae
d) Chlamydia

55. **The longest acting sulfonamide is :** 718

a) Sulfamethoxypyridazine
b) Sulfadoxime
c) Sulfamethaxozole
d) Sulfadiazine

56. **Sulfonamides used for Topical application include all of the following EXCEPT :** 718

a) Sodium sulfadiazine
b) Sodium Sulfacetamide
c) Mafenide
d) Silver sulfadiazine

57. **All of the following are cross-allergenic for a patient sensitive to sulfonamides EXCEPT :** 719

a) Hydrochlorthiazide
b) Acetazolamide
c) Furosemide
d) Diazoxide

e) Procainamide

f) Tolbutamide

58. **The antimicrobial agent which has more antibacterial activity in prostatic and vaginal fluids is :** 720

a) Ampicillin

b) Cephalexin

c) Trimethoprim

d) Sulfadiazine

e) Gentamycin

59. **The combination of Pyrimethamine with sulfonamide is effective in all of the following conditions EXCEPT :** 720

a) Vivax malaria

b) Falciparum malaria

c) Toxoplasmosis

d) Leishmaniasis

60. **Megaloblastic anemia caused by Trimethoprim can be prevented by the simultaneous administration of :** 721

a) Folic acid

b) Vitamin B-12

c) Pyridoxine

d) Folinic acid

e) Ascorbic acid

Reference 2

61. **All of the following drugs are effective in infections caused by Pneumocystis carini EXCEPT :** 1065

a) Co-trimoxazole

b) Pentamidine

c) Clindamycin-Primaquine

d) Amifloxacin

e) Trimethoprim-Dapsone

62. **The drug of first choice for the treatment of Brucellosis is :** 1038

a) Ciprofloxacin

b) Doxycycline-Gentamycin

c) Co-trimoxazole

d) Doxycycline

63. **The fluoroquinolone antibiotic active against anerobic microorganisms is :** 1067

a) Ciprofloxacin

b) Sparfloxacin

c) Ofloxacin

d) Pefloxacin

e) Lomefloxacin

64. **The quinolone antibiotic mainly eliminated nonrenally is :** 1067

a) Pefloxacin
b) Ofloxacin
c) Ciprofloxacin
d) Cinoxacin

65. **The agent commonly used to acidify urine, when methenamine is used as urinary antiseptic, is :**

a) Ascorbic acid
b) Glutamic acid
c) Hippuric acid
d) Pantothenic acid

ANSWERS

54.c 55.b 56.a 57.e 58.c 59.a 60.d 61.d 62.b 63.b 64.a 65.c

ANTIFUNGAL AGENTS

Reference : 2

66. **All of the following antifungal agents are Triazoles EXCEPT :** 1180

a) Econazole
b) Terconazole
c) Itraconazole
d) Fluconazole

67. **The antifungal agent which crosses blood-brain barrier effectively is :** 1180

a) Amphotericin B
b) Clotrimazole
c) Flucytosine
d) Butaconazole

68. **The concentration of Ketoconazole and Itraconazole is reduced by all of the following EXCEPT :** 1181-82

a) Phenytoin
b) Rifampin
c) Ranitidine
d) Food
e) Omeprazole

69. **Bioavailability of which of the following antifungal drug is not significantly altered by food or gastric acidity :** 1183

a) Ketoconazole
b) Itraconazole
c) Fluconazole
d) Amphotericin B

70. **All of the following drugs when given with Terfenadine can cause Torsades de pointes EXCEPT :** 1181-83

a) Fluconazole
b) Ketoconazole
c) Erythromycin
d) Itraconazole

71. **The antifungal drug which acts by inhibiting fungal mitosis is :** 1184
a) Amphotericin B
b) Flucytosine
c) Ketoconazole
d) Griseofulvin

72. **The most effective agent for the treatment of Tinea pedis is :** 1187
a) Econazole
b) Miconazole
c) Tolnaftate
d) Haloprogin

73. **Topical application of antifungal agents is usually not successful for the treatment of :** 1185
a) Onychomycosis
b) Tenia versicolor
c) Tinea capitis
d) Tinea nigra
e) Conditions a and c
f) Conditions b and d

74. **Topical antifungal agent with a broad spectrum of antifungal activity is :** 1186
a) Tolnaftate
b) Miconazole
c) Ciclopirox olamine
d) Haloprogin
e) Naftifine

ANSWERS

66.a 67.c 68.d 69.c 70.a 71.d 72.b 73.e 74.c

ANTIVIRAL AGENTS

Reference 2

75. **The DNA virus which does not utilise host cell RNA polymerase for replication is :** 1191
a) Herpes virus
b) Poxyvirus
c) Adenovirus
d) Papilloma virus

76. **All of the following conditions are caused by DNA viruses EXCEPT :** 1191
a) Small pox
b) Chicken pox
c) Measles
d) Hepatitis B
e) Conjunctivitis

77. **All of the following conditions are caused by RNA viruses EXCEPT :** 1191
a) Rabies
b) Warts
c) Mumps
d) Influenza
e) Yellow fever

Reference 1

78. **The antiviral drug which acts by preventing entry of virus particle into the cell by blocking penetration is :** 730
a) Amantadine
b) Gamma globulin
c) Methisazone
d) Interferons

79. **The antiviral drug which can cause release of catecholamines is :** 731
a) Vidarabin
b) Acyclovir
c) Amantadine
d) Trifluridine

80. **The treatment of choice for Lassa fever is :** 732
a) Vidarabin
b) Acyclovir
c) Gamma globulin
d) Ribavirin
e) Cytarabin

81. **The drug that is effective against Herpes viruses resistant to Idoxuridine is :** 732
a) Cytarabin
b) Trifluridine
c) Acyclovir
d) Ganiclovir

82. **The least toxic and most effective antiviral agent which is a purine and pyrimidine analogue is :** 732
a) Vidarabine
b) Idoxuridine
c) Acyclovir
d) Cytarabin
e) Trifluridine

83. **All of the following drugs have been found to be effective in patients with HIV infection — AIDS or Aids-related complex (ARC) EXCEPT :** 734

a) Zidvudine
b) Didanosine
c) Zalcitabine
d) Acyclovir
e) Stavudine

84. **The antiviral drug that does not require phosphorylation for its activity against Herpes virus is :** 734

a) Vidarabin
b) Foscarnet
c) Acyclovir
d) Ganciclovir

85. **Zidovudine-resistant strains of HIV are susceptible to :** 734

a) Stavudine
b) Acyclovir
c) Didanosine
d) Puromycin

86. **The antibiotic which has been shown to inhibit Poxyviruses is :** 736

a) Doxycycline
b) Chloramphenicol
c) Ciprofloxacin
d) Rifampin

87. **The drug effective in blocking replication of small pox virus is :** 735

a) Gamma globulin
b) Methisazone
c) Interferons
d) Acyclovir

ANSWERS

75.b 76.c 77.b 78.b 79.c 80.d 81.b 82.a 83.d 84.b 85.c 86.d 87.b

ANTI-TUBERCULAR AND ANTI-LEPROSY DRUGS

Reference 1

88. **First line antitubercular drugs include all of the following EXCEPT :** 707

a) Isoniazide
b) Ethambutol
c) Rifampin
d) Rifabutin
e) Pyrazinamide

89. The antitubercular drug which inhibits the growth of tubercular bacilli at an acidic pH is : 710

a) Isoniazid
b) Ethambutol
c) Pyrazinamide
d) Streptomycin
e) Rifampin

90. Advantages of INH as antitubercular drug include all of the following EXCEPT : 708

a) It is effective when taken orally
b) It acts on intracellular bacilli
c) It crosses blood-brain barrier effectively
d) It is bacteriostatic for resting bacilli and bactericidal for dividing bacilli
e) Resistance develops slowly to it when used alone

91. Chemoprophylaxis with INH is indicated in all of the following situations EXCEPT : 708

a) Close contacts of freshly diagnosed cases
b) Pregnant women
c) Persons converting from negative to positive tuberculin test
d) Skin test positive persons with HIV infection

92. Therapeutic indications for the use of Rifampin include all of the following EXCEPT : 709

a) Leprosy
b) Tuberculosis
c) Urinary tract infection
d) Eradication of staphylococcal carriage in the nasopharynx
e) Prophylaxis in contacts of children with H.Influenze type b disease

93. All of the following drugs are bactericidal for tu: ercular bacilli EXCEPT : 710

a) Ethambutol
b) Pyrazinamide
c) Isoniazid
d) Rifampin
e) Streptomycin

94. The drug of choice for suppressing Erythema nodosum leprosum is : 713

a) Dapsone
b) Amithiazone
c) Thalidomide
d) Rifampin

Reference 2

95. Antimicrobial agents with activity against M.Avium complex include all of the following EXCEPT : 1155

a) Rifabutin

b) Clarithromycin
c) Clofazimine
d) Isoniazid
e) Ciprofloxacin
f) Ethambutol

96. **Tubercle bacilli resistant to INH are usually sensitive to all of the following drugs EXCEPT :** 1156
a) Rifampin
b) Ethionamide
c) Pyrazinamide
d) Ethambutol
e) Kanamycin

97. **"Shoulder-hand" syndrome can occur as an untoward effect of which of the following anti-tubercular drug :** 1158
a) Ethambutol
b) Capreomycin
c) Paraaminosalicylic acid
d) Isoniazid
e) Cycloserine

98. **All of the following statements regarding Rifampin are true EXCEPT :** 1160
a) It is well abosrbed orally even in the presence of food
b) It is bactericidal for both intracellular and extracellular organisms
c) Its half-life is progressively shortened during the first 14 days of therapy
d) It imparts orange-red colour to urine, feces, saliva, tears and sweat

99. **Therapy with which of the following drug results in increased urate concentration in the blood :** 1162-63
a) Ethambutol
b) Ethionamide
c) Pyrazinamide
d) Isoniazide
e) Drugs a and c
f) Drugs b and d

ANSWERS

88.d 89.c 90.e 91.b 92.c 93.a 94.c 95.d 96.b 97.d 98.a 99.e

ANTIMALARIAL DRUGS

Reference 1

100. **The antimalarial drug that is active against Hypnozoites is :** 780
a) Chloroquin
b) Primaquine

c) Quinine
d) Quinacrine

101. **The antimalarial drug that renders gametocytes noninfective in the mosquitoes :** 780
a) Primaquine
b) Chloroquine
c) Proguanil
d) Quinidine

102. **An initial loading dose of Chloroquine is necessary because :** 782
a) It is highly bound to plasma proteins
b) It has a long elimination life
c) It is poorly absorbed from the GIT
d) It has a very large volume of distribution

103. **Chloroquine resistance in resistant malarial parasite can be reversed by :** 782
a) Mefloquine
b) Verapamil
c) Quinine
d) Fansidar
e) Desipramine
f) Drugs a and d
g) Drugs b and e

104. **Contraindications to Chloroquine include all of the following EXCEPT :** 785
a) Psoriasis
b) Pregnancy
c) Porphyria
d) Visual field abnormalities
e) Liver damage

105. **The antimalarial drug with longest elimination half-life is :** 785
a) Chloroquine
b) Primaquine
c) Fansidar
d) Mefloquine
e) Proguanil

106. **Contraindications to the use of Mefloquine include :** 786
a) Epilepsy
b) Psychiatric disorder
c) Pregnancy
d) Children under 2 yrs. of age
e) All of the above
f) Situations a and d

107. **Administration of Mefloquine with all of the following drugs is contraindicated EXCEPT :** 786
a) Quinine

b) Propranolol
c) Salbutamol
d) Verapamil
e) Quinidine

108. **All of the following antimalarials can cause hemolysis in patients with G-6-PD deficiency EXCEPT :** 785, 89, 87, 91

a) Chloroquine
b) Pyrimethamine
c) Primaquine
d) Quinine
e) Fansidar

109. **All of the following drugs are effective in the treatment of Chloroquine-resistant Falciparum malaria EXCEPT :** 788, 89, 90, 91

a) Mefloquine
b) Fansidar
c) Proguanil
d) Doxycycline
e) Primaquine
f) Quinine
g) Quinghaosu

110. **The drug of choice for the treatment of severely ill patients with Chloroquine-resistant Falciparum malaria is :** 789

a) Mefloquine
b) Fansidar
c) Quinine
d) Doxycycline
e) Halofantrine

111. **For the treatment of acute attack of Vivax malaria :** 790

a) Quinine is less effective than Chloroquine
b) Quinine is as effective as Chloroquine
c) Quinine is more effective than Chloroquine
d) Quinine is more effective and less toxic than Chloroquine

Reference 2

112. **Rapid-acting blood schizonticides include all of the following drugs EXCEPT :** 967

a) Chloroquine
b) Quinine
c) Pyrimethamine
d) Mefloquine
e) Quininidine

113. **The antimalarial effects of Chloroquine include all of the following EXCEPT :** 970-71

a) It is effective against erythrocytic forms of P.Vivax
b) It is curative for malaria caused by P.Malariae
c) It is curative for transfusion induced Vivax malaria
d) It is effective against gametocytes of P.Falciparum

114. **The most common side-effect produced by Chloroquine in dark-skinned persons is** : 972

a) Headache
b) Pruritis
c) Visual disturbances
d) Nausea
e) Urticaria

ANSWERS

100.b 101.c 102.d 103.g 104.b 105.d 106.e 107.c 108.b 109.e 110.c 111.a 112.c 113.d 114.b

AMEBIASIS AND OTHER PARASITIC INFECTIONS

Reference 2

115. **All of the following drugs are effective in Toxoplasmosis EXCEPT** : 989

a) Fansidar
b) Spiramycin
c) Clindamycin
d) Erythromycin
e) Atovaquone

116. **The antibiotic which has been shown to be effective for Cryptosporidiosis in patients with AIDS is** : 989

a) Paromomycin
b) Spiramycin
c) Co-trimoxazole
d) Erythromycin

117. **All of the following drugs are effective in amebiasis for the treatment of asymptomatic cysts passers EXCEPT** : 991

a) Metronidazole
b) Paromomycin
c) Iodoquinol
d) Diloxanide

118. **The drug of choice for the treatment of late stages of both West and East African Trypanosomiasis is** : 993

a) Suramine
b) Eflornithine
c) Melarsoprol
d) Pentamidine

119. The administration of which of the following drug to leprosy patients can precipitate Erythema nodosum : 995

a) Suramine
b) Atovaquone
c) Pentamidine
d) Fansidar
e) Melarsoprol

120. The Nitroimidazole compound effective in Acute Chaga's disease is : 995

a) Metronidazole
b) Benznidazole
c) Ornidazole
d) Tinidazole

121. Metronidazole is effective in all of the following conditions EXCEPT : 997

a) Symptomatic amebiasis
b) Giardiasis
c) B.Fragilis infection
d) Patients of peptic ulcer infected with H.Pylori
e) Asymptomatic cyst passer infected with E.Histolytica
f) Pseudomembranous enterocolitis

122. Which of the following antibiotic is directly amebicidal : 1004

a) Oxytetracycline
b) Erythromycin
c) Paromomycin
d) Streptomycin
e) Chlotetracycline

Reference 1

123. The antiamebic drug responsible for neurotoxic syndrome SMON was : 796

a) Iodoquinol
b) Metronidazole
c) Clioquinol
d) Oxytetracycline

124. The drug of choice for the treatment of American Trypanosomiasis is : 798

a) Nifutrimox
b) Suramin
c) Pentamidine
d) Benznidazole
e) Melarsoprol

125. All of the following drugs are effective in Pneumocystis Carini pneumonia EXCEPT : 798-9

a) Co-trimoxazole
b) Pentamidine
c) Atovaquone

d) Clindamycin + Primaquine
e) Lincomycin

ANSWERS

115.d 116.a 117.a 118.c 119.e 120.b 121.e 122.c 123.c 124.a 125.e

ANTIHELMINTIC DRUGS

Reference 1

126. **Albendazole is the drug of choice for all of the following EXCEPT :** 805
a) Cysticercosis
b) Hydatid disease
c) Ascariasis
d) Cutaneous larva migrans
e) Intestinal capillariasis

127. **The drug of choice for Fascioliasis (Sheep liver fluke) is :** 807
a) Praziquantel
b) Bithionol
c) Emetine
d) Chloroquine

128. **Diethylcarbamazine is the drug of choice for all of the following EXCEPT:** 807
a) Onchocerciasis
b) Filariasis
c) Tropical eosinophilia
d) Loiasis

129. **Which of the following drug can provoke relapse of malaria in asymptomatic malaria infection :** 809
a) Invermectin
b) Diethylcarbamazine
c) Emetine
d) Bithionol

130. **The drug of choice for Onchocersiasis is :** 809
a) Albendazole
b) Diethylcarbamazine
c) Ivermectin
d) Bithionol

131. **In the treatment of T.Solium infestation, following therapy with which of the following drug, are proglottids expelled intact :** 811
a) Niclosamide
b) Mebendazole
c) Praziquantel
d) Albendazole

132. **Organophosphorus antihelmintic compound, which functions as cholinesterase inhibitor, is :** 812

a) Oxamniquine
b) Invermectin
c) Levamisol
d) Metrifonate

133. **The drug of choice for H.Nana infection is :** 813

a) Niclosamide
b) Praziquantel
c) Mebendazole
d) Albendazole

134. **The drug effective in the treatment of Schistosome infection caused by all the species is :** 815

a) Metrifonate
b) Oxamniquine
c) Praziquantel
d) Mebendazole

135. **Niclosamide is effective in all of the following infestations EXCEPT :** 813

a) Pork tapeworm
b) Beef tapeworm
c) Fish tapeworm
d) Dwarf tapeworm

136. **The drug which causes its antihelmintic effect by producing depolarizing neuromuscular block is :** 817

a) Piperazine
b) Metrifonate
c) Pyrantel pamoate
d) Dichlorophen

137. **Thiabendazole exerts all of the following pharmacological effects EXCEPT:** 818

a) It is the drug of choice for Strongyloidosis
b) It has an anti-inflammatory action
c) It has immunomodulating effect on T cell function
d) It has an analgesic action
e) It possesses an antipyretic effect

Reference 2

138. **Miner's disease and Tunnel disease are the terms used to denote which type of worm infestation :** 1010

a) Ascariasis
b) Hookworm
c) Whipworm
d) Threadworm
e) Pinworm

139. **Which of the following antihelmintic drug can provide complete symptomatic and functional relief in Dracunculosis :** 1011

a) Albendazole
b) Mebendazole
c) Metronidazole
d) Pyrantel pamoate
e) Praziquantel

140. **High incidence of megaloblastic anemia resembling Addisonian anemia is associated with which type of Cestode infestation :** 1011

a) Beef tapeworm
b) Pork tapeworm
c) Dwarf tapeworm
d) Fish tapeworm

141. **WHO report of 1993 indicates that a strong association exists between several forms of neoplastic diseases and :** 1012

a) Ascariasis
b) Taeniasis
c) Schistosomiasis
d) Filariasis

142. **For the treatment of Ascariasis during pregnancy and in children under 2 yrs. of age the drug of choice is :** 1014, 20, 22

a) Mebendazole
b) Albendazole
c) Pyrantel pamoate
d) Piperazine

143. **Diethylcarbamazine exerts all of the following effects EXCEPT :** 1015

a) It causes rapid disappearance of microfilarial forms from human blood
b) It destroys microfilarae of W.bancrofti in a hydrocele
c) It kills worms of adult L.Loa
d) It has little action against adult O.volvulis

144. **Which of the following drug is likely to increase therapeutic and toxic effect of Diethylcarbamazine :** 1015

a) Acetazolamide
b) Ammonium chloride
c) Hippuric acid
d) Mandelic acid

ANSWERS

126.c 127.b 128.a 129.b 130.c 131.b 132.d 133.b 134.c 135.d 136.c 137.d 138.b 139.c 140.d 141.c 142.d 143.b 144.a

ANTI-CANCER DRUGS

Reference : 1

145. **The Gene that has been shown to have mutated from Tumor Suppressor Gene to an Oncogen in a high percentage of cases of several human cancers is :** 823

a) P-60
b) P-53
c) P-24
d) P-70

146. **Cancer chemotherapy can be curative in all of the following disseminated neoplasms EXCEPT :** 824

a) Testicular cancer
b) Hodgkin's disease
c) Choriocarcinoma
d) Colonic cancer
e) Acute lymphoblastic leukemia

147. **Newer classes of drugs that are being developed for the therapy of malignancy include :** 824

a) Inducers of differentiation, intended to form end stage cells with little or no proliferation potential
b) Antimetastatic drugs
c) Hypoxic tumor stem cell-specific agents
d) Tumor radiosensitizing and normal tissue radioprotective drugs
e) All of the above
f) Drugs of type a and d mentioned above

148. **Cell cycle specific antimalignant drugs include all of the following EXCEPT :** 826

a) Mercaptopurine
b) Vincristin
c) Doxorubicin
d) Podophylline alkaloids

149. **Cell cycle nonspecific anti-cancer agents include all of the following EXCEPT :** 826

a) Cyclophosphamide
b) Cisplastin
c) Nitrosoureas
d) Methotrexate

150. **The anti-cancer drug that can cross blood-brain barrier is :** 830

a) Cyclophosphamide
b) Chlorambucil
c) Meclorethamine
d) Carmustin

151. **The Nitrosourea compound which has minimal bone marrow toxicity and is effective in the treatment of Islet cell carcinoma is :** 830

a) Carmustin
b) Streptozocin
c) Lomustin
d) Semustine

152. **The Alkylating agent which can cause disulfiram-like reaction is :** 830
a) Procarbazine
b) Cisplastin
c) Cyclophosphamide
d) Carmustin

153. **The antimalignant drug that can cause hemorrhagic cystitis is :** 831
a) Dacarbazine
b) Altretamine
c) Chlorambucil
d) Semustine
e) Cyclophosphamide

154. **The anti-cancer drug which causes depolymerization of microtubules and mitotic arrest in metaphase is :** 835
a) Procarbazine
b) Cytarabin
c) Vincristin
d) Fluorouracil
e) Mercaptopurine

155. **The broad spectrum anti-cancer drug is :** 837
a) Carmustin
b) Doxorubicin
c) Methotrexate
d) Cisplastin
e) Vinblastin

156. **The anti-cancer drug that causes irreversible, cumulative dose-related cardiac toxicity is :** 837
a) Etoposide
b) Teniposide
c) Vinblastin
d) Doxorubicin
e) Cytarabin

157. **The anti-cancer drug which causes severe or total alopecia at standard doses is :** 838
a) Azactidine
b) Thioguanin
c) Daunorubicin
d) Mitomycin

158. **The drug that is used for Topical intravesical treatment of small bladder papillomas is :** 838

a) Dactinomycin
b) Mitomycin
c) Plicamycin
d) Doxorubicin

159. **The only anti-cancer antibiotic with a cell cycle specific effect is :** 839
a) Doxorubicin
b) Dactinomycin
c) Mitomycin
d) Bleomycin

160. **The anti-cancer drug that can cause fatal pulmonary fibrosis is :** 839
a) Cyclophosphamide
b) Bleomycin
c) Doxorubicin
d) Methotrexate

Reference 2

161. **S-phase specific anti-cancer drugs include all of the following EXCEPT :** 1231
a) Cytosine arabinoside
b) Hydroxyurea
c) Dacarbazine
d) 6-Mercaptopurine
e) Methotrexate

162. **M-phase specific anti-cancer drugs include all of the following EXCEPT :** 1231
a) Vincristin
b) Lomustine
c) Paclitaxal
d) Vinblastin

163. **Which of the following alkylating agent requires biochemical activation before its cytotoxicity becomes evident :** 1234
a) Mechlormethamine
b) Chlorambucil
c) Melphalan
d) Cyclophosphamide

164. **The enzyme responsible for converting Cyclophosphamide into cytotoxic compound is :** 1234
a) Phosphatase
b) Cytochrome P-450
c) Phosphamidase
d) Aldehyde dehydrogenase

165. **The anti-cancer drug that requires initial activation by Cytochrome P-450 is :** 1235
a) Streptozocin
b) Carmustine

c) Dacarbazine
d) Lomustine

166. The Nitrogen mustard which causes less severe thrombocytopenia is : 1238
a) Mechlormethamine
b) Cyclophosphamide
c) Chlorambucil
d) Melphalan

167. The slowest-acting Nitrogen mustard in clinical use is : 1240
a) Cyclophosphamide
b) Melphalan
c) Ifosfamide
d) Chlorambucil

168. The metabolite responsible for causing hemorrhagic cystitis in patients treated with Cyclophosphamide is : 1239
a) Acrolein
b) Phosphramide mustard
c) Carboxyphosphamide
d) 4-hydroxy cyclophosphamide

169. A Flu-like syndrome can occur during treatment with which of the following alkylating agent : 1243
a) Chlorambucil
b) Lomustine
c) Dacarbazine
d) Busulfan
e) Thiotepa

170. Concurrent use of Methotrexate with all of the following drugs can lead to severe myelosuppression EXCEPT : 1246
a) Cisplastin
b) Aspirin
c) Piperacillin
d) Folic acid
e) Diclofenac

171. The agents which have been combined with 5-FU to enhance its cytotoxic activity through biochemical modulation include all of the following EXCEPT : 1250
a) Cisplastin
b) Leucovorin
c) Interferon
d) Methotrexate
e) Pyrimethamine

172. The single, most effective agent for induction of remission in Acute myelocytic leukemia is : 1251
a) Methotrexate
b) Vincristin

c) Cytarabin
d) 6-Mercaptopurine
e) Thioguanine

173. **Purine analogues are used clinically for the treatment of all of the following conditions EXCEPT :** 1252
a) Malignant diseases
b) Immunosuppression
c) Acute gout
d) Chronic gout
e) As antiviral agents

174. **Purine analogue which functions as Adenosine deaminase inhibitor is :** 1257
a) Fludarabine
b) Pentostatin
c) Azathioprine
d) Allopurinol

175. **The drug of choice for Hairy cell leukemia is :** 1257
a) Pentostatin
b) Cladribine
c) Fludarabine
d) Azathioprim

176. **The Vinca alkaloid which has activity against Lung cancer is :** 1258
a) Vinorelbine
b) Vincristin
c) Vinleurosine
d) Vinrosidine
e) Vinblastin

177. **The drug of choice for the curative therapy of metastatic Testicular tumors is :** 1259
a) Vincristine + Bleomycin + Cisplastin
b) Vindesine + Belomycin + Cisplastin
c) Vinblastin + Belomycin + Cisplastin
d) Vinrosidine + Bleomycin + Cisplastin

178. **All of the following anti-cancer drugs can cause the syndrome of inappropriate secretion of ADH EXCEPT :** 1239, 1259
a) Cyclophosphamide
b) Vinblastin
c) Vincristin
d) Busulfan

179. **The drug which acts as inhibitor of mitosis and promotes rather than inhibiting microtubule formation is :** 1260
a) Vinblastin
b) Paclitaxel
c) Cholchicine
d) Vincristine

180. **An antibiotic which functions as an alkylating agent is :** 1268

a) Idarubicin
b) Bleomycin
c) Plicamycin
d) Mitomycin
e) Doxorubicin

181. **Synergestic toxicity results when Methotrexate is used with L-Asparginase provided :** 1269

a) When L-asparginase preceeds methotrexate
b) When methotrexate preceeds L-asparginase
c) When both the drugs are given together
d) All of the above

182. **Intracranial hemorrhage in the first week of therapy can occur following the use of which of the following drugs :** 1269

a) L-Asparginase
b) Mitomycin
c) Cisplastin
d) Hydroxyurea

183. **Which of the following anticancer drug is nephrotoxic and ototoxic :** 1270

a) Doxorubicin
b) Mitomycin
c) Cisplastin
d) Bleomycin
e) Idarubicin

184. **The anticancer drug which has its primary site of action the enzyme Ribonucleosid diphosphate reductase is :** 1271

a) Cisplastin
b) Methotrexate
c) L-Asparginase
d) Hydroxyurea

185. **The anti-cancer drug effective in Polycythemia vera is :** 1271

a) Cisplastin
b) Hydroxyurea
c) Paclitaxel
d) Etoposide

186. **The drug that is of potential benefit in reducing the rate of hemolysis in sickle cell anemia by increasing hemoglobin F formation is :** 1272

a) Mitotane
b) Procarbazine
c) Hydroxyurea
d) Cytarabine
e) Semustine

187. **Hypertensive reactions may result following the use of Sympathomimetic agents or Tricyclic antidepressants, concurrently with which of the following anti-cancer drug :** 1272

a) Procarbazine
b) Dacarbazine
c) Cytarabine
d) Semustine

188. **Which of the following drug can interfere with the adrenal suppression produced by Mitotane :** 1273

a) Triamterene
b) Spironolactone
c) Amiloride
d) Furosemide

189. **All of the statements about Aminoglutethimide, given below, are correct EXCEPT :** 1273

a) It inhibits the conversion of Chloesterol to Pregnenolone
b) Inhibition of Cortisol synthesis by it results in compensatory rise in ACTH secretion
c) Administration of Dexamethasone with it prevents the increase in ACTH secretion
d) It is a potent inhibitor of the conversion of Androgens to Estrogens in extra-adrenal tissues

190. **Which of the following drug is under study as a Chemopreventive in women at risk for developing breast cancer :** 1275

a) Megestrol acetate
b) Diethylstilbesterol
c) Aminoglutethimide
d) Tamoxifen

191. **Match the Agents given in Column A with the Statements given in Column B**

Column A	Column B
1. Leuoprolide	a) Used in Hairy cell carcinoma
2. Flutamide	b) Approved to rescue bone marrow graft failure
3. Interferon Alpha	c) Used for prophylaxis of chemotherapy induced neutropenia
4. Interlukin-2	d) Long acting gonadotropin releasing hormone analogue
5. Granulocyte colony stimulating factor	e) Inhibits translocation of androgen receptor to the nucleus from the cytoplasm
6. Granulocyte/Monocyte colony stimulating factor	f) Useful in kidney cancer

192. **The endocrine treatment of choice for postmenopausal women with metastatic Breast cancer containing ER receptors is :** 1275

a) Hydroxyprogesterone
b) Tamoxifen
c) Aminoglutethimide
d) Diethylstilbesterol

ANSWERS

145.b 146.d 147.e 148.c 149.d 150.d 151.b 152.a 153.e 154.c 155.b 156.d 157.c 158.b 159.d 160.b 161.c 162.b 163.d 164.b 165.c 166.b 167.d 168.a 169.c 170.d 171.e 172.c 173.c 174.b 175.b 176.a 177.c 178.d 179.b 180.d 181.b 182.a 183.b 184.d 185.b 186.c 187.a 188.b 189.c 190.d 191.1=d, 2=e, 3=a, 4=f, 5=c, 6=b 192.b